Imminent Peril

IMMINENT PERIL:
PUBLIC HEALTH IN
A DECLINING
ECONOMY

Edited by
Kevin M. Cahill, M.D.

 The Twentieth Century Fund Press

For Daniel Boyer

Who crosses the barriers of language
and politics to serve his fellow man

RA
445
.I5
1991

Library of Congress Cataloging-in-Publication Data

Imminent peril: public health in a declining economy / edited by
Kevin M. Cahill
   p.   cm.
   Includes bibliographical references.
   1. Medical policy—United States.   2. Public health—Economic
aspects—United States.   I. Cahill, Kevin M.
RA445.I5   1991
363.1'0973—dc20   91-37555
ISBN 0-87078-334-3   : $9.95   CIP

Cover Art: A Board of Health member among cholera victims in New York City in
1854, from the collection of Kevin M. Cahill, M.D.
Cover Design: Claude Goodwin

Published by The Twentieth Century Fund Press
41 East 70th Street, New York, New York 10021

Copyright © 1991 by The Twentieth Century Fund, Inc.
Manufactured in the United States

Foreword

People come together to live; they come together in cities to live the good life. That elevated view of urban life started, as far as we know, with the ancient Greeks and was shared until fairly recently by many Americans.

The city was the crucible of national progress, even of national identity. And the range of human services it offered its residents reflected the richness and diversity of its population. Of course, the underside of the urban environment often was ugly, brutal, and unforgiving. But the idea of progress, of inevitable improvement, was strong. And city dwellers believed in it implicitly. Today, that faith is shaken, in sore need of renewal.

This volume addresses perhaps the critical foundation stone of such a renewal: public health services. Our nation's cities are facing a severe public health crisis. In August, led by Dr. Kevin Cahill, a distinguished group of health professionals and public officials met to examine the state of public health in New York City and by extension other large cities.

The purpose of their efforts is to warn and to guide—to let us know how precarious our public health is, what is wrong with the state of health care in our cities today, and what must be done to avoid a total breakdown of the system. Urban and health issues such as these have long been of concern to the Fund, which supported Dennis Andrulis's *Crisis at the Frontline: The Effects of AIDS on Public Hospitals*, two task forces on the state of New York City, and is now looking at such critical issues as homelessness, access to and long-term health care, and urban poverty.

We are pleased to have been afforded the opportunity to publish this volume of essays. Although this project is a departure from the research and writing projects we manage and operate directly on a range of public policy issues, we are delighted to assist in a modest way in bringing to public attention this lively and provocative discussion of a vital issue.

Clearly, it is imperative that something be done about the public's health. The commitment of our leaders to dealing with this critical issue is evident in the impassioned address of New York's Governor Mario Cuomo, who calls for the federal government to get its priorities straight and spend "on the things that are most important."

We at the Fund believe that spending on the right things is what this nation must do. That is why we have published this volume.

Richard C. Leone, DIRECTOR
The Twentieth Century Fund
September 1991

Contents

Acknowledgments

This book was published six weeks after a symposium had been convened by the Board of Health of the City of New York in late August 1991. Each of the contributors had accepted my invitation to prepare, on less than one month's notice, a substantive paper addressing an obvious public health crisis. Their generosity in participating reflects the importance and urgency of the topic; to each of them I express my profound appreciation.

Many people—and the organizations they direct—helped make both the symposium and this book possible. I wish to thank my fellow members of the Board of Health, Drs. John Cordice, Saul Farber, Pamela Moraldo, and Acting Commissioner Margaret Hamburg, for unanimously endorsing the project. At various stages of this effort, important advice and assistance were graciously provided by Drs. Kurt Deuschle and Kenneth Johnson, and by Majority Speaker Peter Vallone, David Aaron, Peter Presiosi, Joan Durcan, Beverly Goldberg, Patricia Caruso, Robert Schiffer, and Arthur Webb. To each of them I offer gratitude for a job well done. The editing of this manuscript was made both possible and pleasurable because of the heroic efforts of Pamela Gilfond, Senior Editor at the Twentieth Century Fund. Critical practical support was offered by The Twentieth Century Fund, The National League for Nursing, The City Council of New York, The Time-Warner Corporation, and The Tropical Disease Center of Lenox Hill Hospital.

Introduction

❖ *Kevin M. Cahill, M.D.* ❖

The metaphors of the human body come naturally to a physician as he views the ills that plague modern society. Just like patients, cities can rot from within until nothing remains but a hulk artificially maintained by emergency infusions. The signs and symptoms of serious disease are usually obvious, in medical as well as political life—except to those who wish to deny the evidence of steady deterioration and the possibility of death. To those who indulge in such folly, the healing arts offer no immunity. While diagnosis is rarely difficult, devising and administering an appropriate treatment plan can be difficult for both doctor and patient. Cities and states have collapsed before because of benign neglect. Spasmodic efforts at revival are no substitute for a careful, and even courageous, course of therapy. It is important, at least for me in considering public health issues, to maintain that perspective.

We must remind ourselves that all the great city-states in the developed world were created by men and women who desired to live together, sacrificing the security of rural isolation for the stimulation of crowded, noisome towns. They conceived—sometimes motivated by love, sometimes by greed—an urban structure that could sustain their dreams, wild dreams where trade, education, the arts, and political and religious freedoms would flourish in peace and harmony, in an environment that depended upon safe supplies of shared water, food, and even air.

Laws were passed to control pollution for the welfare not only of the individual but of the community at large. In every civilized society, the containment of infectious diseases took priority over commercial gain. The whole concept of quarantine (holding ships in the harbor for forty days) reflected

1

the understanding and acceptance that the public's health stood above all else if a city was to thrive, or even survive.

In his observations on the system of democracy that flourished in this country in the early nineteenth century, Alexis de Tocqueville captured a characteristic American approach in the search for a healthy and safe environment. While emphasizing the individuality of our forebears, he noted their propensity to form civic organizations to guarantee fundamental rights. He wrote: "There is no end which the human will despairs of attaining by the free action of the collective power of individuals.... An association unites the energies of divergent minds and vigorously directs them toward a clearly indicated goal."

Today, there seems to be a steady diminution of that national spirit de Tocqueville so admired, a failure to see beyond immediate, selfish interests, a squandering of the unique heritage of America. The nation seems to have lost its bearings; our priorities have gone awry. Leaders must arrest this drift toward communal disintegration and personal self-destruction. For pragmatic as well as ethical reasons, I suggest this renewal begin with a political focus on public health.

Like de Tocqueville's early pioneers, we must begin our labors convinced that we can overcome the challenges of a harsh new world. I conceived of this book in the belief that even the most intractable problems in this country can be solved if only wise and determined citizens will become involved in helping to define and then to strengthen the necessary political course of action.

There are certainly ominous signs forecasting terrible times ahead for the health of our country unless there is a drastic reorientation of governmental priorities. The world's premier public health system has been pushed toward extinction by draconian budget cuts. Across the land a demoralized professional core of public health workers are trying to cope with an unusual confluence of disparate forces, contending with the emergence of new and the resurgence of old communicable and fatal diseases. The AIDS crisis adds to the chaos by generating confusion, hysteria, and panic—built, at least in part, on ignorance and fear. This ever-changing epidemic has accentuated the ancient clash between individual and public rights, and best demonstrates our current, tragic paralysis in finding solutions at either level.

If we cannot test, if we cannot treat, if we cannot immunize, if we cannot educate, then we shall fall victim to a calamity that will not only fill the corridors of our hospitals but will soon cripple the economic engine, and drive away those precious human resources that give life to cities such as New York. Time is not on the side of those who believe we can continue to replace reality with rhetoric.

The "public" served by the public health system is increasingly the disenfranchised, the uninsured, the impoverished, the homeless, the aged, the addicted. Failing their needs is more than morally indefensible in our "new world order"; it threatens the health of all. For as surely as an untreated tuberculous lesion will cavitate the lungs of a homeless vagrant, so too will the deadly mist of his infection disseminate through every social and economic class, among innocent fellow riders in the subway, or passengers in an elevator and, inevitably, from child to child in the classrooms of our city.

This book offers historical, legal, and field reports that should challenge America's soul. This present crisis must teach us, once again and maybe forever, that no one—no individual, no family, no city, state, or nation—can hope to reach its potential as long as so many are denied their basic rights to public health protection.

Public health programs are not political privileges to be parceled out annually. They must be recognized as fundamental, nonnegotiable prerogatives of every citizen. Such public services must be held immune from those who measure value merely with fiscal scales. There are irreducible levels of health care and prevention that are absolute requirements in the rare system of government our Founding Fathers created.

With an optimism that is necessary to sustain those of us who are privileged to spend our lives amidst dreams as well as sufferings, I have concluded this book with a section on "New Approaches," hoping to draw the best from leaders in both the private and public sectors, unabashedly trying to promote a characteristic that de Tocqueville saw as the essence of America—the willingness to face difficulties together, to make of adversity an opportunity for new thinking, new ways of acting. And if we do it correctly, perhaps we can entice the entire nation, and all its leaders, back to the vision that the good health and welfare of the public is the very foundation of our society. If we were to truly understand this, then never again would public health budgets be gutted, and our efforts would be worthwhile indeed.

The hour for the rebirth of a caring and compassionate country is here, for renewing old priorities that may still allow that rough beast of hope—urban societies with all their failings—to continue, as an Irish poet would have it, slouching toward Bethlehem to be born to a better life.

Part I:

The Foundation

The lessons of history, and the limits defined by legal statutes, are probably the best guides for those empowered by their fellow citizens with decision-making roles in a democratic society. When those judgments deal with life and death, with the protection of the public from imminent peril to their health and welfare, there are, fortunately, numerous precedents and rich traditions on which we depend.

In this section, Professor John Duffy, America's premier medical historian, traces the origins and contributions of Boards of Health in our country. The constitutional basis for public health law is then carefully considered in an eloquent brief by Thomas P. Dowling, Esq.

It is the role of the physician who cares for the sick and dying to translate these tales of the past and rules of the present into a clinical reality, to remind us that health statistics are not merely numbers but human beings. Dr. Margaret C. Heagarty graphically—and with barely controlled outrage—describes the devastation she sees daily in a poverty-stricken, inner-city pediatric service. I provide an analysis of distorted priorities and a faulty budgetary process that almost caused the collapse of a great public health department, and provoked this book.

Assuring Public Health in a Democracy: A Historical Perspective

❖ John Duffy ❖

The prosperity and happiness of any community is determined largely by the health of its people. Where illness abounds and life expectancy is short, the population is neither contented nor productive. Community leaders have recognized this since the dawn of civilization and have taken whatever measures they felt were necessary for the common good.

The rise of cities some six to seven thousand years ago created problems with respect to food, water, and sanitation that could not be dealt with by individuals, thus necessitating community action. With the emergence of nationalism, political leaders began to equate population growth with the nation's strength and the seventeenth and eighteenth centuries saw the emergence of an economic policy known as mercantilism. The mercantilists recognized that health and productivity were closely related—that a healthy population was essential to creating a wealthy and populous state. In consequence, the mercantilists urged political rulers to promote the health and welfare of their subjects. By the eighteenth century, the age of enlightened despots, rulers began establishing what was called a system of medical police.

While governmental supervision of public health in an age of autocracy was designed primarily to benefit the rulers, the underlying assumption—that there was an obvious need for official action to assure community health—was equally valid for the rising democratic states. At a time when the institutionalization of public health was first beginning in America,

Dr. John M. Toner, one of the founders of the American
Public Health Association, speaking before the association
in 1873, declared that the law of nature gives communities
the right to use "an organized medical police," since disease
is calamitous to individuals and "a positive loss to the State."[1]

From the earliest colonial days, American communities sought
to protect the health of their members. Almost from their founding, towns such as Boston and New York employed physicians to provide medical care for the poor, passed quarantine laws, regulated food and water supplies, and sought to
eliminate unsanitary conditions. During the epidemics of smallpox, yellow fever, and other diseases, communities established
pesthouses to isolate the sick, provided medical care, and made
arrangements for the welfare of effected families.

One of the first Americans to urge communal action on behalf
of health was Cadwallader Colden of New York. Colden is
best known for his historical writing and political activities,
but he began his career as a practicing physician. Yellow fever
was threatening New York in the 1740s, and prevailing medical opinion held that epidemic diseases were engendered by
foul miasmas emanating from garbage, human and animal
wastes, and other putrefying organic matter in stagnant
pools and low lying areas. Colden, who was surveyor-general
of the province, stressed that it was the city's obligation to
guarantee the health of its citizens by removing these unsanitary conditions. Spurred on by favorable public reaction to
Colden's appeal, the Provincial Assembly enacted a comprehensive sanitary act applying to New York City. In turn,
the city's Common Council then promulgated a sweeping sanitary code based upon the Provincial law. Enforcement of the
regulations was left to the municipal inspectors; no special
health officers were appointed. New York, however, was still
small, and, in comparison with European cities, it remained
fairly clean until the disruption caused by the Revolution.[2]

New York also remained a relatively healthy city until
the burgeoning population following the Revolution brought

major problems with respect to the city's water supply and the disposal of human wastes and garbage. Still, it was not the rapidly growing sanitary problems but a series of yellow fever epidemics, striking along the Atlantic coast from 1793 to 1806, that served as the impetus for health reform. The first city to suffer was Philadelphia, where the disease killed over 5,000 people within a four-month period. The following year, 1794, the fever appeared in several New England ports, and in 1795 ravaged New York City. Fortunately, New Yorkers had been forewarned by the Philadelphia experience, and a fourteen-man health committee appointed by the governor was given wide latitude to combat the epidemic. Over and above such immediate measures as initiating a massive sanitary program, strictly enforcing the quarantine regulations, and isolating the sick, the health committee recommended the appointment of a permanent Health Office to administer the quarantine laws. In 1796, the state legislature not only accepted this recommendation, but provided a source of income for the Health Office by requiring fees from all incoming vessels.[3]

Cases of yellow fever continued to appear in New York each summer, and, in response to almost 2,000 deaths from a yellow fever epidemic in New York in 1798, a special committee appointed by the municipal council recommended that the city be given wide authority over all matters pertaining to the health and welfare of its citizens. Municipal officers, the report stated, should have such powers as the right to enter and inspect all buildings and grounds; order the removal from the city of any factory, trade, or business that produced "noxious vapors or highly offensive smells"; and require filling and draining of all private land. In an age when garbage collection and street cleaning had been left largely to private initiative, the committee members, well ahead of their time, recommended that the municipality assume full responsibility for these tasks. The committee members also urged that the city construct a municipal water supply and underground sewers.

After citing the many threats to the people's health, the members stated further that they were conscious that their recommendations "must necessarily be productive of much inconvenience to many of their fellow citizens." The report then concluded that the members had "recommended great and strong power to be vested in the Corporation; but they do not believe anything short of it will restore this city to its former healthy state." The city immediately drafted a bill for presentation to the state legislature embodying virtually all of the committee's recommendations. Early in 1799, the legislature enacted the bill into law.[4]

Despite a strict quarantine and an effective sanitary program, yellow fever cases began appearing again late in July 1799. The health committee promptly ordered the evacuation of a number of blocks in the docks' area and provided housing for those dispossessed in the form of tents located on high ground. Since the *Aedes aegypti* mosquito, the vector for yellow fever, has a short range of flight, this policy of mass evacuation worked quite well. Nonetheless, the fever continued to threaten the city in the succeeding years, and, in response to the danger, a new office was created in 1804—that of city inspector. His duty was to report all "nuisances," and prepare drafts of any ordinances "as may be most conducive for the preservation of the health of said City. . . ." The law creating the office also provided for collecting mortality statistics, since the city inspector was given the task of registering the names of all individuals dying within the corporation limits. In January 1805, the city council created a Board of Health, which, with the concurrence of the state legislature, was invested with all the powers relating to public health formerly held by the city council. This first Board of Health, however, was only a temporary agency, appointed on a yearly basis.

Within a few months of its establishment, the Board of Health was faced with fighting the last major yellow fever epidemic to plague New York. The board swung into action as soon as word was received that yellow fever was present in the West Indies: Quarantine and sanitary laws were strictly enforced and preparations were made to care for the sick. When cases were reported in the city, the board again ordered a mass evacuation of infected areas, provided food and housing for the poor who were displaced, and mobilized the city's medical resources. This firm action by the Board of Health, aided by the almost unlimited funds placed at its disposal, minimized the death toll.

In 1819, a few cases of yellow fever were diagnosed, and once again the Board of Health took extraordinary measures, including the removal of all persons from areas infected by the disease. In making the evacuation announcement, the board first explained its reasons for the order and then added: "Measures of precaution, when attended with present inconvenience, are always unpalatable, and they usually become more so, when most completely successful. It frequently happens that their failure is received as their best justification."[5]

In 1828, shortly before the first of three epidemics of Asiatic cholera to sweep through America in the nineteenth century, the Board of Health issued a pamphlet describing its organization, powers, and duties. The board's main duty, the pamphlet declared, was to prevent the spread of disease and to exercise all powers that "the public good shall require." The appearance of cholera cases late in June 1832 brought a renewed effort to cleanse the city, to establish temporary hospitals, and to take other measures to reduce the impact of the disease and alleviate human suffering. Instead of the customary July 4 celebrations, the holiday was proclaimed a day of fasting and prayer.

By the time of the second cholera epidemic in 1849, the intellectual climate had changed. In reaction to President Zachary Taylor's proclamation of August 3 as a national day of fasting and prayer, the editor of the *Daily Tribune* responded that cholera, rather than a punishment from God, was "the natural result of our violations of the Physical Laws of the

Universe." The solution, he wrote, was to discover which laws man had broken and correct the situation. As with yellow fever, nothing was known of the cause or cure of cholera. All the Board of Health could do was to enforce the quarantine and sanitary laws and help the sick and dying.[6]

The enormous expansion of New York City in the antebellum period, brought about by the opening of the Erie Canal in 1825 and the waves of impoverished immigrants that poured into the city in the 1840s and 1850s, led to much inefficiency and corruption. Even worse, since an arithmetic increase in population seems to result in an almost geometric increase in sanitary problems, health conditions steadily deteriorated.

The middle decades of the nineteenth century saw the beginning of the early sanitary movement in the United States, with middle- and upper-class reformers campaigning in nearly every city for better water and food supplies, improved garbage collection and sewer systems, and the removal of all hazards to health. In New York, throughout the 1850s, the Association for Improving the Condition of the Poor and the New York Academy of Medicine fought for health reform with little success. Fortunately for their cause, in 1859 the New York Sanitary Association was organized. This association drew into its ranks a wide range of professional and business leaders, including nearly all members of the Academy of Medicine's Committee on Public Health.

Still, despite collaborating with the Academy of Medicine and the Association for Improving the Condition of the Poor, the Sanitary Association was unable to overcome opposition from entrenched Tammany Hall politicians. Late in 1863, a new and broader organization, the Citizens' Association, was formed. Realizing the need to create public awareness of the city's extremely poor health conditions, the association sent a circular/letter to physicians requesting their help. In response, a large number of doctors met and organized a Special Council for Hygiene and Health, a body that included such leading health reformers as Drs. Joseph M. Smith, Stephen Smith, Willard Parker, Elisha Harris, and Alfred C. Post.

While the Citizens' Association was campaigning for a municipal health program, the Council on Hygiene and Health undertook a street-by-street survey of health and sanitation in the poorer areas. The results of this survey, published in June 1865, revealed such atrocious health conditions that the state legislature was shocked into passing the Metropolitan Health Act of 1866, a law that created the first effective city health department in the United States.[7]

The Metropolitan Health Act was shaped largely by Dorman B. Eaton, who is best known for his work with the United States civil service law. Due largely to his efforts, the Metropolitan Board of Health was given exceedingly broad powers. Section 12 of the law transferred all powers "for the purpose of preserving or protecting life or health, or preventing disease" to the board. The board could order owners or occupants of property to rectify sanitary conditions or to cease and desist from any actions considered a threat to community health. In enforcing its actions, the board could call upon the police or use its own officers for this purpose.[8]

Shortly after the formation of the board, the members issued a pamphlet in which they pledged "to perform their duty without fear or favor." While preferring voluntary cooperation, the board declared that it intended "to exert its powers to the utmost," for the health law was "founded on the theory that individuals have no right to peril the lives of thousands; [and] that the poor have a right of protection against avarice and inhumanity." Recognizing that many of the board's actions were arousing opposition, the second annual report declared: "The Health Department of a great commercial district which encounters no obstacles and meets with no opposition, may safely be declared unworthy of public confidence; for no sanitary measures, however simple, can be enforced without compelling individuals to yield something of pecuniary interest or of personal convenience to the general welfare."[9]

In the spring of 1866, Asiatic cholera once again became pandemic, spreading across Europe and threatening America. The Board of Health, aware that the city's sanitary conditions were deplorable, began taking the usual quarantine and sanitary precautions. As the threat from cholera increased, the board announced, on April 13, that a state of imminent peril and danger existed. To meet the danger, the board resolved to undertake a massive sanitary program, to assume responsibility for caring for the sick and burying the dead, and to request the authority to spend whatever funds were required, and, if necessary, to borrow additional money. The request was approved by Governor Fenton and the state of emergency was officially proclaimed on April 24. At that time, many of the lowest economic class, those most subject to cholera, lived in foul, damp cellars, made even worse by drainage from the omnipresent privies. The board, acting on legal advice, began a policy of evacuating the inhabitants of the worst of these dwellings. At the same time, not without difficulty, it made arrangements to remove and house passengers from ships detained in quarantine, and to separate the well from the sick.

Even before the first case of cholera appeared, the Board of Health, in conjunction with the New York Academy of Medicine, had organized a corps of physicians and nurses to care for the sick, designated certain hospitals for cholera patients, and established a highly coordinated system of medical care using six city dispensaries as bases. Whenever a case of cholera was reported, the visiting physician would determine whether to treat the patient at home or send him to one of the temporary hospitals. In some cases, an entire household was evacuated and the premises cleaned and disinfected. In addition, a prompt house-to-house survey was undertaken to be sure no cases were missed. A special disinfectant depot and laboratory was established, and disinfectant squads were maintained on a round-the-clock basis to clean and disinfect any premises where cholera had been reported.

By the time the epidemic ended, at a cost of almost six hundred lives, the Board of Health had removed thousands of residents from unsanitary basement dwellings, mobilized the city's doctors and nurses, undertaken a massive sanitary program, and spent approximately a quarter of a million dollars, an immense amount in that day. Compared to the ravages of most nineteenth century epidemics, New York came off lightly in 1866, and the actions of the Board of Health won for it the gratitude and respect of New Yorkers.[10]

When Asiatic cholera threatened once again in 1892, the board promptly took decisive steps to ward off the disease. By this date, the role of the cholera bacillus was understood, and the board instructed the commissioner of public works to inspect the Croton watershed (the main source of New York's water supply), ordered its food and milk inspectors to be "especially vigilant," and had the Sanitary Department carefully inspect approximately forty thousand tenement houses. Some years earlier, a summer corps of fifty physicians had been established to work during the months of July and August, visiting tenement homes with infants or children. In view of the threat from cholera, the summer corps was kept in operation during the fall months, thus temporarily adding fifty physicians to the department's permanent corps of medical inspectors. Pamphlets were issued in various languages informing the public of the nature of cholera and urging personal hygiene. The number of Health Department ambulances used to remove contagious disease cases to the hospitals was increased from three to nine, and the Disinfecting Corps was strengthened. In September, responding to developments in bacteriology and the urging of Dr. Herman A. Biggs, a new Division of Pathology, Bacteriology, and Disinfection was established. Happily, the board's prompt action managed to keep the disease at bay, and only nine deaths from cholera were recorded.[11]

The next emergency facing the Board of Health arose in 1907, when a justifiable strike by the city's garbagemen left piles of refuse accumulating in warm weather. As the situation worsened, the Board of Health assumed control of street cleaning, assigning its sanitary superintendent, Dr. Walter Bensel, to head the city's Street Cleaning Department and mobilizing workers from its own department and elsewhere to remove the garbage. Under Bensel's direction, the Street Cleaning Department was reorganized and the practices that had outraged the garbage workers were removed. By November, with the situation under control, the Health Department returned the operation of street cleaning to regular city officials.[12]

Early in June 1916, cases of poliomyelitis began appearing in New York. On June 30, as reports of cases began increasing, the United States Public Health Service was notified. Polio had been a reportable disease in the city since 1910, but the disease had been of negligible proportions. By late June, polio was spreading rapidly and arousing great public apprehension. As with the great plagues of the nineteenth century, the disease was of mysterious origin, could kill or cripple its victims, and proved most deadly to children.

Faced with this mortal and crippling disease of unknown origin, the Health Department decided on a policy of full publicity and education. On July 2, the Board of Health declared a state of great and imminent peril. All July 4 celebrations were canceled, and children were prohibited from attending motion picture theaters. On August 10, when 5,652 cases had resulted in 1,260 deaths, Dr. Haven Emerson, the health commissioner, announced that the opening of schools, scheduled for September 11, would be delayed until October. On August 31, Acting Mayor Frank Dowling requested an appropriation of $250,000 to care for polio patients discharged from the contagious wards.

By this date, the number of new cases was beginning to fall, and on September 21 the Board of Health announced that schools would open on September 25. Despite strong opposition from the League of Parent's Associations, the Health Department held firm on the date. Dr. Emerson declared that he would "bear full responsibility for anything that happened as a result of the opening of the schools." As a concession to apprehensive mothers, the school superintendent stated that the attendance law would not be enforced.

The epidemic was declared over on October 31. A final summary showed that between June 1 and October 31 some 9,023 cases had resulted in 2,448 deaths. In reviewing the epidemic, Dr. Emerson wrote that this was the first occasion when a consistent campaign of publicity and education had been undertaken during the course of an epidemic. The department had required compulsory notification of all cases, and either the hospitalization of patients or else their quarantine in "sanitized" homes.

As had been the case in earlier epidemics, private physicians were mobilized to work with the department's staff in conducting house-to-house visits in infected districts in search of cases. Understandably, with a strange and fearful disease, when newspapers reported that an experimental procedure was being tried—one consisting of injecting new patients with serum from the blood of recovered patients— a number of mothers on the East Side, fearful that blood would be taken from their children, sought to hide the presence of new cases. This problem was not unique to New York; many immigrants in all major American cities, wary of any kind of official, had fought to prevent their children from being vaccinated for smallpox or from being taken away to hospitals for contagious diseases. In a final comment, one with a familiar ring, Dr. Emerson stated that many private physicians temporarily lost their entire practices for taking care of polio cases.[13]

While the occasions when the Health Department declared a state of imminent peril had invariably redounded to its credit, the reverse was true in February 1946. A strike of tugboat workers in that month shut off fuel supplies to the city. Mayor William O'Dwyer, on conferring with his various commissioners and the Office of Defense Transportation, was assured that a fuel shortage was inevitable. On February 7, he issued an emergency proclamation to this effect. Five days later, Health Commissioner Ernest L. Stebbins declared a state of imminent peril. The weather was exceedingly cold with heavy snow, and fearing that lack of fuel for utilities and heating would create serious problems, Stebbins promptly ordered industries to start closing down.

The Board of Trade and businessmen in general were so outraged that the emergency proclamation was withdrawn the next day, and pressure was brought on the mayor to dismiss Stebbins. As an elected official, Mayor O'Dwyer was in a difficult position, but he publicly defended Stebbins until former Mayor Fiorello La Guardia criticized the health commissioner in a radio address. Shortly thereafter, according to Stebbins, the mayor told him to leave office immediately. In view of his information, Stebbins acted correctly, but it turned out that the Office of Defense Transportation had underestimated the city's fuel reserves. As a result, a good health commissioner was forced from office, and the Health Department was discredited.[14]

With the exception of the tugboat strike, during which the Health Department went beyond its normal sphere and relied upon statistics from an outside agency, the occasions when the Health Department used its extraordinary powers to declare an emergency situation were those when the need was obvious. Epidemics of Asiatic cholera and yellow fever were so terrifying and deadly that scarcely anyone questioned the actions of the health authorities. The polio epidemic of 1916 also fell into this category, and Health Department action during the garbagemen's strike in 1907, which left huge piles of garbage festering in the streets under the hot summer sun, scarcely needed justification.

Today, the threats to public health are much more subtle, but not necessarily any less dangerous. Pollution of air and water present both short- and long-range threats; elaborate food processing and distribution methods require constant supervision; an unequal medical care system has left thousands of women in the lower economic groups without prenatal care and their children with little or no medical attention; any relaxation of vaccination efforts to eliminate traditional killer diseases of children can be disastrous; and in many other ways the wary eye of the Health Department is essential to the proper functioning of an urban society.

Preventive medicine, the major function of a health department, is highly cost effective. The success of polio vaccines eliminated the need for staffing and maintaining thousands of iron lung machines and prevented the disabling of many thousands of individuals. Maternal and child care programs, a major responsibility of all health departments, shared a good part of the credit for the reduction in infant mortality and the growth of healthy children during the past one hundred years. In a day when we are once again emphasizing individual responsibility for health—through campaigns advocating exercise, sound diet, and the practice of safe sex, as well as seeking to discourage the use of tobacco and drugs—it is well to remember that seventy years ago, health departments were teaching children to wash, bathe, and clean their teeth, while public health physicians and nurses were carrying the lessons of personal and public hygiene to their parents. Then as now, preventing illness was infinitely less costly than caring for the sick and disabled.

The value of preventive medicine can readily be seen in comparing the death rates from diphtheria, scarlet fever, whooping cough, and measles within the past century. In the last three decades of the nineteenth century, the annual deaths from diphtheria in New York City rarely fell below 1,000; on three occasions, they numbered over 2,000. In the peak year, 1894, a total of 2,359 children died from the disease. Scarlet fever deaths in the same period averaged close to 1,000 per year, with the death toll reaching 2,000 on two occasions. Measles caused the death of about 700 children a year, and whooping cough annually killed another 300 to 500. But thanks to the introduction of vaccines, in 1950, the city, with a much larger population, had only 2 deaths from diphtheria, and two years later, the Health Department reported that for the first time in history no deaths from whooping cough had occurred, and that for the third successive year no fatalities had resulted from scarlet fever.[15] While deaths from measles were sharply reduced in the first half of the twentieth century, success against the disease awaited an effective vaccine in the 1960s.

Although these disorders, as with a number of others, are no longer a major concern, any relaxation of vaccination programs for infants and children opens the way for renewed epidemics. The introduction of vaccination in the first two decades of the nineteenth century drastically reduced the terrible epidemics of smallpox. By the 1830s, as remembrances of this terrible pestilence faded from public memory, vaccination was neglected, and the disease began flaring up, peaking in a series of major epidemics in the Civil War and postwar years. Fortunately, the emergence of public health agencies and mass vaccination drives brought smallpox under control by the early twentieth century. Yet as late as 1900, twelve Tulane University medical students caught smallpox; three of whom died. The revival of measles in the past several years serves as a reminder that eternal vigilance is not only the price of safety, it is also the price of public health.

An authoritarian society has one advantage over democracies: the ability to establish a sound public health policy by decree. Some sixty years ago Dr. Fred Lowe Soper of the Rockefeller Foundation was commissioned by President Getúlio Vargas to eradicate the *Aedes aegypti* mosquito from Brazil. Backed by a presidential edict authorizing his mosquito inspectors and teams to enter all homes and businesses,

Soper effectively carried out his assignment. With the backing of the Pan American Health Organization and the Latin American governments, he carried the eradication program all the way north to the southern border of the United States. In America, public health is primarily in the hands of states and local governments, and its citizens firmly believe in private property and individual rights. Neither state legislatures nor Congress is willing to grant any agency carte blanche authority to enter and search all homes or premises. On these two rocks, Soper's hope of eliminating the *Aedes aegypti* mosquito from the Western hemisphere foundered, and within a few years the mosquito had gradually reinvaded the Latin American countries.[16]

The importance of health education should not be underrated. One of the great success stories in this area has been the campaign against smoking started by the Surgeon General's Report on Smoking and Health in 1964. Nonetheless, health education, which is quite possibly the most essential

Another story, that of Mary Mallon, better known as Typhoid Mary, illustrates how the task of public health officials has been made more difficult in recent years—this time by the emphasis upon civil rights. Early in this century, Mary Mallon was diagnosed as a typhoid carrier. After she was found responsible for several typhoid outbreaks, she was warned not to accept employment as a cook. When she repeatedly disregarded these warnings and caused further outbreaks (Americans have great faith in making a law, but they have little hesitancy in disregarding the same law if it seems inconvenient or unnecessary), the Health Department, on its own authority, had her placed in confinement until she died in 1938.[17] In contrast, in today's society, in which civil libertarians have forced hospitals to release thousands of mentally ill patients (who now constitute a large percentage of the homeless) and vociferous citizens still oppose vaccination, health departments must rely more than ever upon health education.

function of a health department in a democracy, is still only one part of public health. The threats to community health arise from many sources. A reduction in spending for preventive medicine inevitably means much greater costs in the future in terms of medical care and in the loss of productivity and quality of life.

The Role of the Law in Public Health

❖ *Thomas P. Dowling, Esq.* ❖

The role of the law in matters of public health is a venerable and powerful one, having its roots in the ordinances and proscriptions of ancient governments, rulers, and creeds. Dietary restrictions on the consumption of parasite-prone meat, the confinement to leprosariums, the regulation of prostitution, and the management of inoculations are found in the earliest annals of recorded history, reflecting the ancient maxim: *Salus populi suprema lex*—the welfare of the people is the supreme law.

The Romans enacted public health laws guarding aqueducts from pollution, mandating the inspection of sewer systems, requiring the destruction of contaminated foodstuffs, and regulating brothels, burial grounds, and public baths.

In colonial America, epidemics of smallpox and yellow fever sparked a succession of health ordinances, but urban public health measures were already in place, regulating in New Amsterdam, for example, such diverse activities as the disposal of refuse, the construction of privies, the slaughter of beef and swine, the quality of bread, and the constraint of unfettered hogs.

One decree promulgated in 1658 in this city, provided that:

> WHEREAS many, even the greatest part of the burghers and inhabitants of this City build their privies even with the ground with an opening towards the street, so that hogs may consume the filth and wallow in it, which not only creates a great stench and therefore great inconvenience to the passers-by, but also makes the streets foul and unfit for use, therefore. . . the Burgomasters and Schepens herewith order and command, that all and everybody . . . shall break down and remove such privies coming out upon the street.[1]

These ordinances were only fitfully observed, even when buttressed with the use of informers. In his *History of Public Health in New York City 1625-1866*, Professor John Duffy reports a succession of citizen complaints during the years of Dutch and English rule, followed by the enactment of still more ordinances aimed at abating these same unsanitary conditions. Some of these complaints came from observant individuals who saw an association between yellow fever and marshy and swampy ground, fetid pools of water, and other conditions of poor drainage, leading them to urge the enactment of corrective sanitary measures. How close they were to the real cause.

Quarantines and evacuations were more vigorously enforced, but they could only mitigate the damage. Urban inhabitants lived in constant fear of pestilence—including yellow fever, smallpox, malaria, and cholera.

Government response to these epidemics of the eighteenth century typically involved ad hoc actions by local municipalities, which appointed "health officers" or "health committees," often delegating to them authority to deal with the crisis through quarantine and evacuation.[2] It came to be gradually recognized, however, that a body with competence in public health was needed on a permanent basis.

Thus, in 1805, New York City, pursuant to enabling legislation passed by the State, created the New York City Board of Health and delegated to it considerable power, including the right to quarantine and to levy fines up to $1,000. One of the board's early acts, recounted in Professor Duffy's history, was to order the evacuation of what is now the Wall Street financial district in an effort to combat the yellow fever epidemic of 1805.

Massachusetts established state and local Boards of Health in about 1869. The orders of one local board, that in Cambridge, set the stage for a confrontation between the imperatives of public health and the United States Constitution.

Pursuant to authority delegated by a Massachusetts statute,[3] the Board of Health of the City of Cambridge, on February 27, 1902, adopted a regulation providing that:

> Whereas, smallpox has been prevalent to some extent in the city of Cambridge, and still continues to increase; and whereas, it is necessary for the speedy extermination of the disease that all persons not protected by vaccination should be vaccinated; and whereas, in the opinion of the board, the public health and safety require the vaccination or revaccination of all the inhabitants of Cambridge; be it ordered, that all the inhabitants of the city who have not been successfully vaccinated since March 1st, 1897, be vaccinated or revaccinated.[4]

One Henning Jacobson refused to be vaccinated; he was charged in a criminal complaint and arraigned. He pleaded not guilty and was tried by jury, urging in his defense that the compulsory vaccination regulation:

> . . . was in derogation of the rights secured to the defendant by the 14th Amendment of the Constitution of the United States, and especially of the clauses of that amendment providing that no state shall make or enforce any law abridging the privileges or immunities of citizens of the United States, nor deprive any person of life, liberty, or property without due process of law, nor deny to any person within its jurisdiction the equal protection of the laws.[5]

The trial court refused to so instruct the jury, which returned a verdict of guilty. Jacobson was sentenced by the court to pay a fine of $5 and stand committed until the fine was paid.

In his appeal to the Supreme Judicial Court of Massachusetts, the judgment below was affirmed. In construing the ordinance, the appellate court made certain findings that, ninety years later, still have relevance in debates over the use of vaccines:

... for nearly a century most of the members of the medical profession have regarded vaccinations, repeated after intervals, as a preventive of smallpox; that, while they have recognized the possibility of injury to an individual from carelessness in the performance of it, or even in a conceivable case without carelessness, they generally have considered the risk of such an injury too small to be seriously weighed as against the benefits coming from the discreet and proper use of the preventive. . . .[6]

Jacobson appealed the affirmance to the United States Supreme Court in *Jacobson v. Massachusetts*,[7] where Justice Harlan expressed the question as follows: "Is the statute, so construed, therefore inconsistent with the liberty which the Constitution of the United States secures to every person against deprivation by the State?"[8]

In addressing that issue, the Court acknowledged the preeminent role that public health occupies in the spectrum of government activities:

> The authority of the state to enact this statute is to be referred to what is commonly called the police power,— a power which the state did not surrender when becoming a member of the Union under the Constitution. Although this Court has refrained from any attempt to define the limits of that power, yet it has distinctly recognized the authority of a state to enact quarantine laws and "health laws of every description;" . . . According to settled principles, the police power of a state must be held to embrace, at least, such reasonable regulations established directly by legislative enactment as will protect the public health and the public safety.[9]

Speaking for the majority, Justice Harlan also validated the delegation of the state's powers to boards such as the Board of Health of the City of New York (which, by this time, was one hundred years old):

> It is equally true that the state may invest local bodies called into existence for purposes of local administration

with authority in some appropriate way to safeguard the public health and the public safety. The mode or manner in which those results are to be accomplished is within the discretion of the state, subject, of course, so far as Federal power is concerned, only to the condition that no rule prescribed by a state, nor any regulation adopted by a local governmental agency acting under the sanction of state legislation, shall contravene the Constitution of the United States, nor infringe any right granted or secured by that instrument.[10]

The conflict to be resolved between these public health imperatives and the individual's constitutionally guaranteed rights was underscored by the Court's portrayal of the defendant's position:

We come, then to inquire whether any right given or secured by the Constitution is invaded by the statute as interpreted by the state court. The defendant insists that his liberty is invaded when the state subjects him to fine or imprisonment for neglecting or refusing to submit to vaccination; that a compulsory vaccination law is unreasonable, arbitrary, and oppressive, and, therefore, hostile to the inherent right of every freeman to care for his own body and health in such way as to him seems best; and that the execution of such a law against one who objects to vaccination, no matter for what reason, is nothing short of an assault upon his person.[11]

These powerful words, in defense of which rivers of blood have been spilled, would in many debates carry the day, but not with such worthy an adversary as the commonweal.

In balancing these competing and compelling claims, the Court rejected the notion that constitutional rights are absolute, observing that a "Society based on the rule that each one is a law unto himself would be confronted with disorder and anarchy."[12]

In responding to the allegation that the statute was unreasonable or arbitrary, the Court declared:

The authority to determine for all what ought to be done in such an emergency must have been lodged somewhere or in some body; and surely it was appropriate for the legislature to refer that question, in the first instance, to a board of health composed of persons residing in the locality affected, and appointed, presumably, because of their fitness to determine such questions. To invest such a body with authority over such matters was not an unusual, nor an unreasonable or arbitrary, requirement. Upon the principle of self-defense, of paramount necessity, a community has the right to protect itself against an epidemic of disease which threatens the safety of its members.[13]

In words often heard in more recent debates over the value of fluoridation, the risks of inhaling second-hand smoke, and other health controversies, the Court also addressed challenges to the efficacy of the vaccination, holding that such was in the province of the legislature not the court and that, in any event, its efficacy was a belief widely held by both the public and the medical profession:

While not accepted by all, it is accepted by the mass of the people, as well as by most members of the medical profession. It has been general in our state, and in most civilized nations for generations. It is generally accepted in theory, and generally applied in practice, both by the voluntary action of the people, and in obedience to the command of law. Nearly every state in the Union has statutes to encourage, or directly or indirectly to require, vaccination; and this is true of most nations of Europe. . . . A common belief, like common knowledge, does not require evidence to establish its existence, but may be acted upon without proof by the legislature and the courts. . . . The fact that the belief is not universal is not controlling, for there is scarcely any belief that is accepted by everyone. The possibility that the belief may be wrong, and that science may yet show it to be wrong, is not conclusive; for the legislature has the right to pass laws which, according to the common belief of the people, are adapted to prevent the spread of contagious diseases.[14]

Before affirming the judgment of the Court below, the Supreme Court felt constrained to express a caveat that is as apt today as it was in 1905:

Before closing this opinion we deem it appropriate, in order to prevent misapprehension as to our views, to observe—perhaps to repeat a thought already sufficiently expressed, namely—that the police power of a state, whether exercised directly by the legislature, or by a local body acting under its authority, may be exerted in such circumstances, or by regulations so arbitrary and oppressive in particular cases, as to justify the interference of the courts to prevent wrong and oppression. Extreme cases can be readily suggested. Ordinarily such cases are not safe guides in the administration of the law.[15]

Jacobson v. Massachusetts affirmed, in 1905, the power of the law to both invoke (through legislation) and enforce (through the courts) public health measures. It is still the law. It validates (as do the express terms of the New York City charter) the actions of the Board of Health, and its teachings are still instructive in addressing the manifold and perplexing public health problems that we struggle with today and that we must confront with wisdom and determination.

Suffer the Little Children: A View from the Trenches

❖ Margaret C. Heagarty, M.D. ❖

I write to bear witness, to tell the sorry tale of the lives of children of many parts of this grand city. And I long for the talent of a great novelist or painter, for the story of these children deserves such genius. The testimony I give comes from my personal experience, for you see, for the past dozen years I have worked in Harlem on the seventeenth floor of the Harlem Hospital where I direct the department of pediatrics. The children I will try to describe are not statistics, not anonymous abstractions to me, rather they and their families have names and faces, problems, strengths, aspirations, tragedies. And while I am going to tell you about the parents and children of Harlem, the story I tell can be replicated in any low-income neighborhood in this city or in other major cities in this nation.

Central Harlem is a community of about 100,000 people, roughly 90 percent of whom are black and the remainder largely Hispanic. About 25,000 children, 23 percent of the population, live in the community. They are poor; more than two-thirds receive public assistance. Their educational levels are very low; only about one-third can read at grade level. The unemployment rate is more than double the national average, and almost one-third of adolescents are unemployed.[1]

The Harlem Hospital Center is the major source of medical care as well as the single largest employer in the community. The staff of the department of pediatrics, in its

I wish to express my profound gratitude for the collaboration of David Bateman, M.D., Chief of Neonatology, Harlem Hospital Center, and Assistant Clinical Professor of Pediatrics, College of Physicians & Surgeons, Columbia University.

wards and clinics and with its five neighborhood family-care centers, together with three New York City Department of Health child-health stations, provide the pediatric care for most of the children in the area.

For many years, the children of Harlem have lived in deprived, dangerous, and depressed circumstances, but in the past ten years, their lives, indeed their very survival, has been placed in question.

Figure 1 shows the percentage of low birth weight infants born at the hospital over the past several years. Note that in about 1986, this percentage, always well above the citywide average, increased sharply. These trends are not peculiar to Harlem. In 1989, the citywide percentage of low birth weight was at a level of 9.7 percent, a 14 percent increase over the past five years. The percent of women who deliver infants at the hospital, but who have not received prenatal care, runs about 15 percent. Since low birth weight is the major cause of death in infants under one year of age, it is not surprising that the New York City infant mortality rate also increased from 12.8 per thousand in 1986 to 13.3 per thousand in 1989. Central Harlem has the highest infant mortality rate in the city, almost twice the rate for the entire city.[2]

Predictably enough during this time, the hospital's neonatal intensive care unit became stretched well beyond its capacity. Figure 2, which shows the average daily census of this unit, is merely a symbol of what has happened to the city's perinatal care system over the past few years. There have been times in the recent past in which there wasn't a free neonatal intensive care bed to be found in the city, in either public or private hospitals.

During this same period, the city's neonatologists faced the reappearance of syphilis, a nineteenth century disease, thought to have been conquered with the discovery of penicillin. Unfortunately, pregnant women who contact syphilis, if untreated, can infect their newborns with the disease. Figure 3 shows that the rate of congenital syphilis in infants born

Figure 1
Percent of Low Birth Weight Infants*

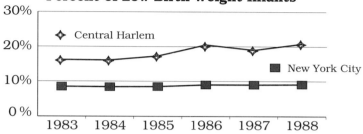

Source: New York City Department of Health

*Birthweight less than 2,500 grams

Figure 2
Harlem Hospital
Neonatal Intensive Care Unit

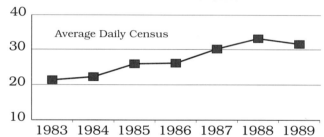

Source: Harlem Hospital Newborn Service

Figure 3
Cases of Congenital Syphilis

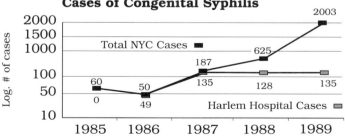

Source: Harlem Hospital Newborn Service and
New York City Department of Health

at the Harlem Hospital escalated sharply in the late 1980s. Indeed, the pediatricians of my department have cared for infants with congenital syphilis of a type that hasn't been seen since my father was in practice in the 1930s. These data simply reflect the very serious syphilis epidemic in New York City since the mid-1980s.

Several events have caused this deterioration in the health of newborns and children. For example, while many in New York City experienced considerable economic prosperity during the 1980s, the poor got poorer. The "poverty" income level for a family of four calculated in 1966 constant dollars decreased 18.3 percent, or from $3,317 to $2,711 in the period between 1966 and 1990.[3] The number of people receiving some form of welfare increased by 87.5 percent in the twenty-five years since 1966, while the number of children on public assistance increased by 51.3 percent.[4] And as the poverty of families and children of many of this city worsened, with very few in authority seeming to notice or care, a new tyrant appeared on the streets of Harlem and other disadvantaged neighborhoods. About 1986, a new cheap form of cocaine—crack—suddenly appeared to attack the young men and women of these communities. In great measure, the increase in low birth weight, infant mortality, and probably syphilis is the result of this new insult to the poor.

Figure 4 shows the dramatic increase in the number of newborns reported by the Harlem Hospital department of pediatrics to the New York City Child Welfare Administration—one of the sadder results of the cocaine epidemic. This epidemic has produced huge numbers of displaced infants and children, for whom the city's Child Welfare Agency must assume responsibility because their parents are addicted to crack/cocaine. While we have some early evidence that the crack epidemic may be abating somewhat, by June 1991, New York City has almost fifty thousand children in foster care, many of them children of parents involved in drugs—usually crack/cocaine. By June 1992, the New York City

Human Resources Administration predicts that another five thousand children will enter the foster care system.[5] Think of it. Fifty thousand is larger than the population of my home town in West Virginia. It is larger than the population of Scarsdale or Larchmont. A small city of displaced poor children, legions of lost children whose lives have been seriously damaged, perhaps forever.

But the crack epidemic has brought other forms of pain and suffering to the children of Harlem and other disadvantaged communities. For while urban low-income communities have always been dangerous for children, crack brought with it a level of violence that had never been seen before. Figure 5 shows the number of children under the age of

Figure 4
Substance Abuse Allegations
New York City Child Welfare Authority

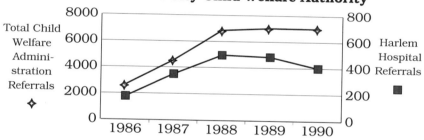

Source: New York City Human Resources Administration, Harlem Hospital Newborn Service

Figure 5
Gunshot/Stab Wounds in Children
Harlem Hospital Admissions

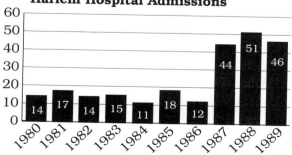

Source: Harlem Hospital

sixteen who were admitted to the Harlem Hospital because of gunshot or stab wounds. Suddenly, in 1987, the number of these admissions increased four times—all the result of the crack epidemic. At times in the past few years, my wards have looked more like a MASH unit, a casualty station, than a pediatric inpatient service. From 1983 to 1987 in the city, half the deaths of children due to injury were the result of violence. Guns caused half of these violent deaths.

As the chemical virus, crack, was appearing in the low-income communities, another lethal biologic virus was also showing its face. Over the decade of the 1980s, we have all been forced to confront the entirely new viral infection AIDS. As the AIDS epidemic spread, it has increasingly attacked our low-income communities. Figure 6 gives a picture of pediatric AIDS in Harlem, as seen by the number of Harlem Hospital admissions of children with the disease over the past several years. About 1.5 percent of pregnant women in this city are infected with this virus, and most of them are poor minority women, who were either infected through their intravenous drug use or who have had contact with an HIV-infected drug using man. In some areas of the city, the prevalence of the AIDS virus in pregnant women is as high as 3 percent to 4 percent. About 30 percent of the infants of these women are infected and will develop the disease. Over the

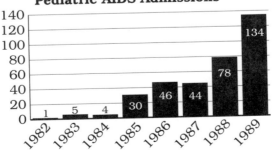

Figure 6
Harlem Hospital
Pediatric AIDS Admissions

Source: Harlem Hospital

next decade, as many as forty thousand children may become orphans because their parents have died of AIDS.

But the story of the poor child does not end with low birth weight or syphilis or crack or violence or AIDS. There is more. In the past decade, as the affluent of the city enjoyed the fruits of leveraged buy outs (whatever they were), the fruits of playing with stocks and bonds, many of our poor lost their homes, lost that most fundamental need: shelter. And those without shelter were not just the mentally ill, the alcoholic; they were, and are, women and children, whole families. On any given night, 7,900 children sleep in one of the city's shelters.[6] By our indifference or by our impotence, whatever the reason, we in New York, as in other cities in this nation, have created a new class of urban refugees—women and children, homeless—living in refugee camps we call shelters. Certainly not places one calls home.

We should therefore not be surprised that the city now faces epidemics of the classic diseases of poverty and over-crowding—nineteenth century diseases medical science conquered thirty years ago. In the past two years, thousands of poor African-American and Latino children have had measles. Last year, almost 2,500 children were reported with the disease, and by May of this year, about 3,100 cases of measles had already been reported to the Department of Health.[7] Since measles has been a preventable disease for more than twenty-five years, this epidemic is simply another example of our indifference and unwillingness to do what we already know how to do, for the children of our city. But not only has measles reappeared, in these same communities the rate of tuberculosis has reached epidemic proportions. In tandem with the increased number of adults with tuberculosis, now five times the national rate, the number of children with the disease, as reported by the Department of Health, rose by 97.3 percent from 1989 to 1990.

But as the 1980s came to a close, the Bonfire of the Vanities did indeed occur, for the financial sky fell upon New York

City. As near as I can determine, along about the time Mayor Dinkins decided to run for office, something terrible happened to the city's economy and we entered a perhaps predictable serious economic recession. And so for the past year or more, those concerned with the city's children have fought a rear guard action to try to maintain the limited services available for them.

For example, in the department of pediatrics of Harlem Hospital alone, the budget for professional services has been reduced by 7 percent to 8 percent. That means that Harlem now has three fewer pediatricians than it did a year ago. In late July, more than a hundred people—technicians, security guards, dietary aides—were "laid off" from the hospital, and a week later another twenty-plus administrative personnel were fired. And the hospital still faces a $9 million "problem," to use the current euphemism for a deficit. Where in the world the hospital is going to find $9 million is a mystery. Unless the hospital simply closes something big. But what to close? The clinics, inpatient units? Should I reduce the staff and size of the neonatal intensive care unit? Maybe I should close the clinic for adolescents or the primary care neighborhood clinics. But even if I close something, I will be forced to reinvent it, because I have no choice. Public general hospitals are hospitals of last resort. They can't and shouldn't turn any child away. There must always be room in our Inn. So despite the obvious increased morbidity in the city's poor children, the municipal hospital system responsible for most of their care is slowly but inexorably hemorrhaging.

But not only direct medical services are in jeopardy. The New York City Department of Health, which is traditionally responsible for many services for children— maternity services, school health, child health stations, immunization and lead poisoning programs—has also been seriously affected by these current budget reductions. When the dust finally settled after the City Council and mayor decided on this year's budget, the school health program was cut by 50 percent.

Translated to reality, in the coming year, a team of two nurses and one aide will be responsible for the thirty or forty schools in a school district. And the child health clinics, which provide as much as 15 percent of the primary care for the city's poor children, have also been affected. During the past fiscal year, 1990, more than thirty-eight positions were left unfilled, causing a reduction of about twenty thousand visits for more than six thousand children. So much for the strategy of budget freezes and attrition. We should not be astonished that we have a major measles epidemic.

These financial decisions have spared no aspect of the city's child-care system. Almost $24 million have been taken from the Human Resources Administration's children's programs. A reduction of more than $2 million in the Child Welfare Administration of the Human Resources Administration, the agency responsible for child protection and foster care, will result in such changes in the work load of case workers as to risk placing many children in considerable jeopardy.

As I have pondered these calamities to services for children, I have wondered what to do. The first very human reaction is to look around for someone to blame, to scapegoat. I could, of course, as many do, blame the poor themselves. I have noticed recently a growing conservative rhetoric, which, in stressing personal and family responsibility, has a certain ring of "blame the victim." And there is always government to be blamed. But I have come to the conclusion that Pogo is correct: "We have met the enemy and they are us." With our representative form of government, our political leaders give us what most of us say we want. And what most of us want is not to pay for it—certainly not by increased taxes for services for children or for anything else for that matter.

So if we have only ourselves to blame for the problems of services for children, what should we do? First and most obvious, those in authority, with influence, and I don't just mean our political leaders, must convince the rest of us that the problems of poor children are real. Without using excessive Irish hyperbole, I believe that if we don't soon intervene to save this generation of urban poor children, we risk a crisis that makes the threat of Saddam Hussein look like child's play. We must convince the body politic that the dangers of inaction, of indifference to these children, are more serious than any real or imagined foreign threat to the country.

Second, we must do what we know how to do. We must have the resources to take the traditional public health measures necessary to protect the children's as well as the public's health. In our panic about our economic problems, we must not destroy the city's system of public health. We must not permit the loss of child health clinics that will administer the immunizations that would prevent such epidemics as measles. We must have the ability to find the cases of tuberculosis. We must have a viable school health program to do the screening examinations, administer immunizations, and locate children with serious health problems. These are simple things. We know how to do them. We have known how to do them for ninety years.

Third, we must advocate fundamental reform of the medical care system. The time has long since come for the nation to deal with the problem of the thirty-seven or so million citizens in this country without access to medical care simply because they have no way to pay for it. The public hospital system of this city must rely upon city tax levy funds to subsidize medical care for the large number of citizens among us who have no health insurance. In the best of times, city hospitals are underfunded, embattled institutions. In times of economic recession like these, the ability of the city to pay for the medically indigent becomes even more problematic. But my department must provide care for all children who come to us, whether they have insurance or not. It is simply not acceptable for us not to have the basic requirements to do this job.

Fourth, in coping with the serious human, social problems of many of these children and their families, we must be prepared to reexamine old premises and to encourage innovation and new ways of providing services. As a nation, we don't seem to mind spending huge amounts of money on mechanical widgets, astronomical sums for experimental gadgets that may or may not work, space stations, supersonic airplanes, and space telescopes. But when confronted with the complicated human problems of our fellow citizens, we throw up our hands. Phrases like "We can't throw money at the problem" or "They are our permanent underclass, who cannot be helped" are usually heard in these debates. Yet if we are to intervene in the cycle of poverty for the urban child, we must begin a "Star Wars" program for children.

The mayor's recently announced Family Preservation Initiative, which will give families in danger of losing children to foster care intensive preventive services, is such an innovation. But given the talent of this city, other innovations are doubtless available. A greatly enhanced day-care program for poor infants and preschool children, which would place them in safe and stimulating environments for much of the day, might be considered. The grandmothers of our urban disadvantaged communities are very nearly exhausted. It is they upon whom the care of the offspring of their drug-addicted children has fallen. Perhaps some methods giving them some support and respite as they take up this burden should be developed. And finally, the capacity for drug treatment must be expanded immediately. Drug users must have access to drug treatment on demand. And since crack/cocaine addiction in such large numbers is a new phenomenon, new strategies and treatments for this addiction should be considered.

Careful evaluations must accompany the development of new strategies and programs to deal with these new problems of children. But we should not worry so much if some of them don't work or if some of them don't work for everyone. If we don't mind spending money on widgets that turn out not to work so well, then we shouldn't mind spending a little money on social interventions that are not all spectacular successes.

At the turn of the last century, New York City was a glittering place, a time of Diamond Jim Brady and Lillian Russell, of the unimaginable wealth of the Robber Barons, a time when the wonderful mansions that still line Fifth Avenue were built for the affluent upper class. But the city had its dark side in the ghettos of the Lower East Side, in which the poor, the recent immigrants from Europe, were to be found. A hundred years ago, the poor were Irish and Italian and Polish, German, Jewish. The children suffered from malnutrition, tuberculosis, measles, other epidemic diseases. Their parents, many of them, numbed the pain of poverty by addiction to alcohol. But a hundred years ago, this city had a group of talented and determined people—Jacob Riis, Lilian Wald, the muckraker journalists who could and did tell the story of that generation's children in a way that could and did move the larger community to take action to protect and defend them.

Those caring people were determined to make certain that the poor children of their time survived and flourished. Now the endangered children are not European, but African-American emigrants from the South, who came to escape economic and racial oppression; they are Hispanic, from Puerto Rico, the Dominican Republic, the Caribbean Islands, Haiti. But all of them have come to this city for the same reasons our ancestors did a century ago. They are as surely our brothers and sisters, our children, as those others were one hundred years ago. To deny them what they need to grow and develop and to enter the mainstream of our city's life is to deny our heritage. In simple justice, we must do what that earlier generation did for us; for we all are immigrants, boat people. The measure of our own success gives us a debt we dare not fail to repay. It is our moral obligation.

Averting Disaster: A New York City Case Study

❖ *Kevin M. Cahill, M.D.* ❖

Early June 1991 may have been the nadir of government support for public health in the city of New York. A set of unusual circumstances led to the near-destruction of the oldest and finest Department of Health in the United States of America. The official New York City executive budget, slated for adoption before July 1, 1991, had slashed the department's personnel by 25 percent. One quarter of the skilled health workers, staffing vital programs that protect the welfare of all New Yorkers, were to be fired. How this almost came to pass, and what was done to avert disaster, holds important lessons for all other cities and states that may face similar fiscal crises.

The exact extent of state support for New York City services, normally known by April 1, varied widely and wildly throughout the spring of 1991. The state executive and legislative branches were mired in a bitter war of words, producing no solid financial estimates on which the city could plan. The shadow of the Financial Control Board and the overt suspicions of municipal unions further complicated the normal budgetary process, fostering an atmosphere in which self-interests and even fears of survival flourished. The vulnerable are, inevitably, the first victims of such political battles. Spokesmen for the weak in our society were shamefully absent or silent in the spring of 1991.

To provide a balanced budget, all New York City agencies had been asked to prepare program and personnel options to satisfy specific percentage reductions. If undue hardship was to be expected, the mayor's office had inaugurated a two tier safety net system through which affected agencies could appeal to the first deputy mayor for exemptions and, ultimately, to the mayor for emergency relief.

The Department of Health negotiations were handled by the commissioner. His management style was one of extreme isolation and insulation. He involved none of his deputy commissioners in the full negotiating process, each having been asked to address only his or her specific area of concern, each encouraged not to discuss the ongoing budget negotiations either within or outside the department. This approach prevented the normal flow of information and healthy pressures that are essential to all dispute resolutions. This official policy of silence undoubtedly contributed to the striking absence of concerned comment from medical and health-oriented organizations, institutions, and academies that should have been vigorously supporting the existing, important programs of an obviously threatened department. The only major constituent groups to actively promote its cause during the negotiating period were those concerned with AIDS.

In late spring, the commissioner abruptly resigned his position, leaving a vacuum in which no one else was fully conversant with essential details of a budget that would shortly devastate the health services of the city. Health was the only agency in city government not to have filed an appeal, and this failure was painfully reflected in the final executive budget. In retrospect, it is clear that the normal process of budget negotiations simply did not take place in 1991 for the New York City Department of Health.

The priorities of any government can be found in its executive budget. Here the political promises finally fade and, particularly in an era of limited resources, society's value judgments are translated into specific allocations. As governor of New York, Franklin Delano Roosevelt stated in 1928: "The test of our progress is not whether we add more to the abundance of those who have much, it is whether we provide enough for those who have too little." One of his predecessors, Al Smith, was even more direct, saying: "Let's look at the record."

The standards of humanism in the 1991 record were but a faint shadow of the noble traditions and patterns of New York's past. While the Department of Health personnel were cut 25 percent, *the largest layoff proposed for any city agency*, the Department of Transportation and its meter maids were reduced by a fraction of 1 percent, with similar protection for the income-generating divisions handling law and economic development, city planning, buildings, and investigations. The security services—police, fire, and probation—were deemed "sacrosanct" and immune from significant personnel cuts. The perils inherent in an impending health emergency, the threat of an unchecked disease spread, did not provoke similar consideration from those responsible for the welfare of the city. The dye had been cast with scarcely a ripple of dissent.

On June 11, a new acting commissioner of health was appointed. With the executive budget scheduled for final adoption later that month, she reviewed the fiscal plan she inherited—a plan adopted almost by default—with growing dismay. She immediately notified several members of the Board of Health and, with the endorsement of my colleagues on the board, the following letter was sent to the mayor on June 18.

June 18, 1991

The executive budget for the Department of Health poses the type of peril to the public safety for which the New York City Board of Health was initially created. The board has the legal and moral obligation to call such dangers to the attention of the mayor, the City Council, and the public, and to encourage all such necessary actions as may be required to protect those most in need.

The Board of Health was not consulted in any of the discussions leading to the budget reductions accepted by the recently resigned commissioner of health, despite the fact that many of the cuts would require amending the existing Health Code (a prerogative of the board and not the Department of Health). If the executive budget cuts are implemented without change, one can confidently predict an explosive spread of disease, suffering, and death. I list below only some of the cuts accepted by the department:

1. Eliminate the entire school health and immunization programs; to give some indication of the public health seriousness of this action it should be noted that last year over 100,000 inoculations against measles were provided to school children. To eliminate that service in the midst of the worst nationwide measles epidemic in decades is, in my judgment, a violation of law as well as common sense.

2. Eliminate all mental health and dental services, and radically reduce the nighttime medical coverage, for the entire New York City prison population. If the level of violence in our prisons is now frightening, imagine inmates denied help with painful dental abscesses or psychotic crises.

3. Eliminate the entire bureau that serves Families with Special Needs; these programs offered essential services to those with serious physical handicaps as well as to the homeless. One must question the fundamental priorities of a Health Department that accepts a budget with a 60 percent reduction in family health services and disease intervention.

4. Eliminate the Division of Day Care and Day Camps. The Health Code has been strengthened, in recent years, in order to guarantee that these centers are run in a safe manner and by qualified personnel, preventing, as one example, those with a history of sexual abuse from working in such facilities. This effort, now to be abandoned, had been made to assure the safety and welfare of innocent toddlers.

5. Eliminate the Drug Treatment Program for Pregnant Mothers; this seems to be an almost inconceivable rejection of the most vulnerable unborn, assuring a dramatic rise in addicted babies and many unnecessary infant deaths.

6. Cut the world-renowned Department of Health Laboratory by 50 percent, and thereby drastically reduce the ability to diagnose every communicable disease from HIV infection to tuberculosis and syphilis. This proposed cut would not only result in devastating delays reporting critical lab tests, but would have a horrendous impact on the Poison Control Centers that annually save so many children's lives.

7. Cut the Bureau of Lead Poisoning by 50 percent, assuring, for future generations, mental tragedies in inner-city children. This cut involves an issue of deep concern to the Departments of Housing and Education as well as Health.

8. Cut the services for diagnosing and treating sexually transmitted diseases among the poor by 30 percent—again an action taken in the midst of a massive epidemic of these infections.

9. Reduce the work force of the Department of Health *by the largest percentage of any city agency.* Surely this distorted sense of priorities must not go unquestioned. Granted that fiscal crises demand sacrifices, there seems to be no logic in virtually destroying a department devoted to protecting life by preventing disease. The skills and expertise of health and laboratory workers require years of training and are in high demand in the private sector; devastating a carefully nurtured team that cannot be replaced is simply poor management.

Many of these proposed eliminations or reductions in services are in areas where legal mandates exist, and to pursue such cuts will inevitably result in the loss of various state, federal, and Medicaid grants. I believe that many of the proposed cuts are of questionable legality, are imprudent and violate the fundamental traditions that once made a caring New York a beacon for those tired, hungry, poor masses who built, and continue to build, our society.

The Board of Health of the City of New York is unique in our governmental system in that it has been empowered with distinct legislative and administrative, as well as advisory, duties. No other board functioning under the New York City Charter can override the decisions of a commissioner, amend, alter or revoke applicable codes, establish rules and regulations, impose fines, and, in the "presence of great and imminent peril to the public health," the Board of Health can *order* the department "to do such acts beyond those duly provided for the preservation of public health, including the power to take possession of and occupy as a hospital any building or buildings in the city, as the board, in good faith, may declare the public safety and health to demand."

These "extensive powers" are not new. The first Board of Health was established in 1805 when the City Council and the mayor authorized the board to hold hearings and investigations, and supervise the paid employees of the city in all matters that relate to the public's right to health and the prevention of disease. Throughout the nineteenth century most health "emergencies" came from the legitimate fear of epidemic diseases, and the board used its powers on many occasions to stem the spread of yellow fever, cholera, and typhoid by various quarantine measures. The board was not expected to wait until an epidemic erupted to treat illnesses; ideally, it used its powers to prevent disease. Even in the present era the emergency powers of the board continue to be invoked to prevent expected health problems that could result from garbage strikes or explosions which contaminated areas with asbestos.

In normal times the board traditionally defers to the directions of the commissioner of health, but the power to assume leadership is available and can—and should—be used in emergency times. At present there is a predictable health crisis impending. There is a long and rich body of specific statutes as well as binding tradition that demand the board "exercise all the powers that the public good shall require," especially when there is an "imminent peril" to the "neglected, dying poor," to infants and children, and where infectious and communicable diseases are certain to spread.

The proposed budget cuts will inevitably invite a health crisis and it would be a violation of law as well as good conscience for this Board of Health not to speak out clearly for the public welfare.

Sincerely,

Kevin M. Cahill, M.D.
Senior Member
The New York City Board of Health

The mayor, the speaker of the City Council, the corporation counsel, the acting commissioner, and their staffs then worked in consultation with the Board of Health and succeeded in restoring the majority of the funds cut. Our joint actions effected a substantial, though still insufficient, budgetary adjustment for a single year—a gratifying but short-term political gain. A battle had been won, not the war.

The long-term objectives of the Board of Health are to inform and educate the citizens and their elected representatives that basic public health services are essential if the city is to remain viable, and to protect the public from imminent

Department of Health
Fiscal Year 1991 Adopted Budget
Total Department of Health Budget – $327,188,735

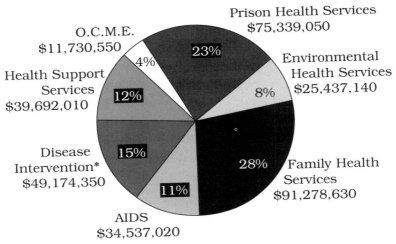

O.C.M.E.
$11,730,550

Health Support
Services
$39,692,010

Disease
Intervention*
$49,174,350

AIDS
$34,537,020

Prison Health Services
$75,339,050

Environmental
Health Services
$25,437,140

Family Health
Services
$91,278,630

*Disease Intervention excludes AIDS

Source: New York City Health Department, budget document, April 1991

peril when a health emergency threatens their welfare. Looking back from the brink, it is clear that public health programs are very vulnerable, particularly in a declining economy. To help avoid future disasters, here as well as in other municipalities across the country, one might draw the following conclusions from the recent New York City experience:

1. Health threats that are beyond the scope of any individual or physician to handle have been recognized, from the very origins of civilized society, to be the responsibility of government. Leaders in both government and the private sector must be reminded of the importance of public health in preserving our cities, our states, and their economies. They must be more understanding of, and ever vigilant in, protecting these essential programs.

2. Elected officials and the public at large must better appreciate that those who most fully rely upon public health services are often incapable of arguing for their needs and their

Department of Health
Fiscal Year 1992 Executive Budget
Total Department of Health Budget – $243,221,389

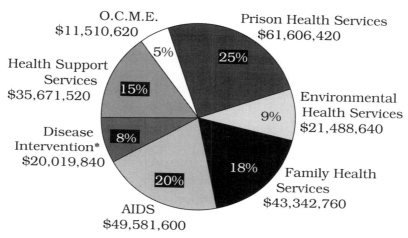

O.C.M.E.
$11,510,620

Prison Health Services
$61,606,420

Health Support
Services
$35,671,520

Environmental
Health Services
$21,488,640

Disease
Intervention*
$20,019,840

Family Health
Services
$43,342,760

AIDS
$49,581,600

*Disease Intervention excludes AIDS

Source: New York City Health Department, budget document, April 1991

rights. In the current New York City case study, the executive budget recommendations posed an obvious imminent peril to the homeless, the poor, infants, children, high-risk pregnant women, and prisoners—to name but a few of the vulnerable groups utterly dependant on government for their health care and protection. It must also be clearly understood that the budget cuts, if enacted, would have exposed all New Yorkers, regardless of social or economic class, to those communicable diseases that rapidly spread in any urban setting.

3. The internal government budget process should never be dependent on a single individual. In this instance, an unusual, isolated management style perverted the normal democratic process and almost proved destructive to the department. The resignation of the commissioner left no single deputy aware of the totality of impending cuts.

4. The appeal process should never be based on the failure of a single individual to activate the system.

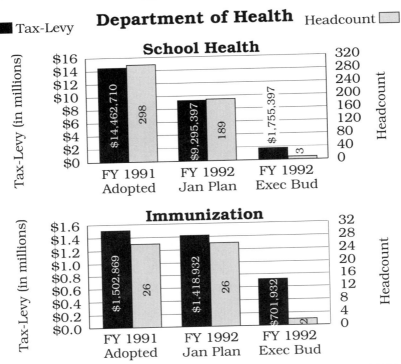

Source: New York City Health Department, budget document, April 1991

5. There must be a greater appreciation of the skills that public health workers possess, and of the obvious fact that their talents are eagerly sought in the private sector. Once professionals leave public jobs for the better pay and nicer surroundings of the private sector, it is unlikely they will ever return to government work. Cutting 25 percent of a trained department staff was a shortsighted, self-destructive management decision.

6. The Board of Health and/or a citizen equivalent body must be involved throughout the budget negotiating process in order to assist governments in making the wisest choices when allocating scarce resources.

7. Other concerned constituencies should be more actively involved in offering their suggestions and advice during the budget process.

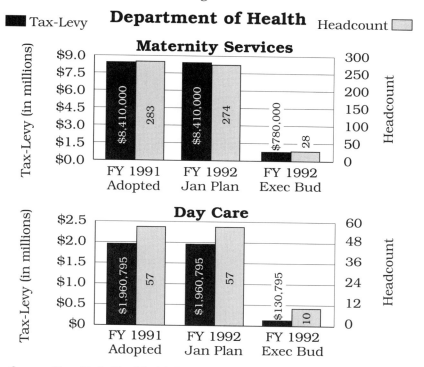

■ Tax-Levy   **Department of Health**   Headcount □

Source: New York City Health Department, budget document, April 1991

8. Elected officials must be aware, especially in a declining economy, of the danger of allocating limited funds largely on the basis of political pressure or the popularity of a particular disease. In the executive budget, for example, AIDS funds were expanded while family services, disease intervention, pest control, lead poisoning, immunizations and school health programs (to name but a few) were drastically cut. These critical value judgments should have been recognized as such by political leaders and more openly discussed before final decisions were made.

9. We must continue to seek definitions of those non-negotiable parameters and irreducible levels of public health services through conferences such as this.

Part II:

The Economics of Public Health

Economic realities often limit our best intentions. The dreams and goals of local governments, just as those of individuals, families, and businesses, are ultimately shaped by monetary considerations. Elected officials annually try to produce balanced budgets, allocating finite public resources that attempt to satisfy the almost infinite demands of the citizenry. It is an exercise that requires wisdom and compassion as well as fiscal skills. In determining public policy, financial arguments may be more persuasive than moral condemnations or appeals to charity or decency.

In this section, the extraordinary economic demands of the AIDS epidemic are seen by Dr. David Rogers as national responsibilities that cannot be assumed within a traditional local public health budget. Dr. Marianne C. Fahs details the long-term costs of cutting public health programs, demonstrating the folly of such a transient expedient. Finally, projecting current health expenditures into the next generation, James Jones and Deborah Steelman, Esq., offer a scenario that is virtually insupportable unless greater public/private cooperation and imagination become the norm in America.

The Special Case of AIDS in Public Health

❖ David Rogers, M.D. ❖

These are bitter times for anyone truly concerned about public health. In New York City, emergency rooms and intensive care units are overflowing, and the percentage of emergency-room patients admitted for inpatient care has risen substantially. There have been dramatic increases in tuberculosis, sexually transmitted diseases, and drug-exposed births. Medicaid costs are rising rapidly. Health-care personnel are in short supply. Draconian cuts in the financing of day care, pediatric dentistry, maternal health services, screening for lead poisoning, and public health education threaten to dismantle the foundations of preventive health care. Superimposed on this bleak portrait is the major epidemic of our century: AIDS and HIV infection.

We are in the midst of a public health disaster of monumental proportions, a disaster all the more tragic for its preventability.

We know that if we immunize children they do not get measles. Yet we had two thousand cases of measles in New York City last year. We know that if we provide education about HIV transmission, if we treat drug abuse, and teach addicts to use clean needles, HIV infection rates can be slowed. Yet they continue to soar nearly unchecked among New York City's drug abusing population.

It must be that we have chosen not to prevent these disasters. Some people argue that we do not have enough money to do everything, and other things must take precedence. I submit that we *do* have enough money but simply are not willing to fund public health adequately. We have enough money to meet the cost of routine health care; we have

enough money to pay for extraordinary burdens like AIDS;
we even have the money for new, innovative public health
initiatives.

Earthquakes and floods are not preventable, usually not
even predictable. But we find the money to meet the emergency needs they pose. By contrast, our public health failures
are predictable and preventable. We do nothing to prevent
them, and we do not even provide disaster relief. Currently,
public health in general, and AIDS in particular, are in a state
of protracted emergency need.

The cost of the choices we have made, in economic terms
alone, is staggering. In the case of AIDS, our shortsighted,
inadequate funding for prevention has meant that the United
States spent an estimated $5.8 billion on treatment for peo-
ple with HIV infection in 1991. In 1992, these costs are
expected to rise nearly 24 percent, and about 20 percent per
year for at least two years thereafter. Fortunately, with
advances in clinical treatment of symptomatic AIDS and
expensive new drugs for prophylaxis, people with AIDS
live longer. Unfortunately, given also the greater numbers of
AIDS patients with substance abuse and other serious medical problems prior to infection, the projected lifetime cost for
an HIV infected person is now about $85,000.

In New York State, more than $1.1 billion in federal, state,
local, and private money was spent in fiscal year 1990-91 on
medical, social, and support services for HIV-infected people. The total bill for that year, including prevention programs,
testing, epidemiology, research, planning, and administration, was $1.4 billion, 29 percent higher than the previous year.

Even these enormous sums are not disaster relief. Combined
federal and state spending does not provide adequate services to those infected and has barely begun to stem the
rate of new infections.

There are not only more patients with AIDS; they are
poorer. When the count is finished, Medicaid costs for
persons with HIV/AIDS in 1990 in New York State are

expected to exceed $500 million, an 85 percent increase in just two years.

A few more facts to put this into perspective:

❏ As of July 31, 1991, there were almost 187,000 cumulative cases of AIDS (as defined by the Centers for Disease Control) reported in the United States. By the end of 1993, between 390,000 and 480,000 cases are projected.

❏ New York State, the center of the HIV epidemic in this country with nearly 40,000 cases of CDC-defined AIDS to date, has 21 percent of the U.S. total and almost as many cases as all of Europe.

❏ While the growth rate of new AIDS cases has slowed, projections estimate that New York State will see more new cases of AIDS in the next five years than have occurred in the past decade. Between 150,000 and 250,000 of the one million or more people infected with HIV in the United States are in New York.

❏ In New York State, blacks and Hispanics account for 61 percent of the total number of AIDS cases, 82 percent of AIDS cases in women, 88 percent of pediatric AIDS cases, and 82 percent of drug injectors with AIDS.

❏ For the past several years, IV drug use has been the leading risk factor for AIDS in New York State. New York's 45 percent of total cases with an IV drug use risk factor is more than twice the proportion in U.S. cases.

❏ Women are the fastest growing group of AIDS patients in New York State.

❏ New York City has more cases of CDC-defined AIDS than the next four highest U.S. cities combined (Los Angeles, San Francisco, Houston, and Washington, D.C.).

❒ The AIDS incidence in New York City's least affected neighborhood is twice the national average.

❒ AIDS is now the leading cause of death among New York City men age 25-49 and New York City women age 20-39.

New York's health professionals, hospitals, and public health services are sorely stressed. Time is running out to break the back of this epidemic. But during a fiscal crisis can we spend what is needed on AIDS and still fund other essential public health programs? The answer we have been getting is no, that we must reduce school immunization programs or prenatal care in order to fund AIDS. That is nonsense.

AIDS is in many respects a disaster outside the realm of standard public health issues. The magnitude of the epidemic, its rapid spread, infectious nature, and scientific complexity, its concentration among the young, and its enormous impact on the health-care system make it as virulent a threat to health planning as it is to those at risk of infection.

But while AIDS is a unique and monumental crisis, it cannot be separated from the other major health and social problems of our time. It is impossible to design programs to detect and treat AIDS without directly confronting issues like drug abuse, sexually transmitted diseases, tuberculosis, lack of access to primary care, family disintegration, and our reluctance to provide services for people whom we do not like.

Many AIDS patients are drug-using parents and their children, crack addicts and alcoholics, adolescent and adult prostitutes, the uninsured, the homeless, and the mentally incompetent. AIDS is exacting an exorbitant toll in disenfranchised and minority communities already beset by poverty, violence, and poor health. These are all issues that we must address if we are to be a viable nation.

AIDS does not need a larger share of a public health pie that is too small to feed the nation. The nation needs a larger public health pie. In this time of reassessing priorities and defining goals in the post-cold war era, we must decide that the health of our population is vital and that we are willing to pay for it.

If we do not choose to fund decent health care for all people, if we do not choose the obvious economic benefits of preventing rather than treating disease, if we cannot see AIDS as a catastrophe that supersedes our normal health-care needs and planning apparatus, then we have seriously circumscribed our public health responsibilities.

Lately it seems that the federal government is ready to abdicate these responsibilities. After finally recognizing the need for a more appropriate response to the AIDS epidemic, the federal government sabotaged AIDS disaster relief to be provided through the Ryan White Care Act. Of the $880 million approved by the House and Senate, only one-fourth ($220 million) was actually granted. Only $144 million of that was new money. At best, only a small additional sum can be expected. The act was passed overwhelmingly with great fanfare, but the evisceration was done very quietly.

This is extraordinarily cynical conduct. Ten years after recognition of the HIV epidemic, we are still waiting to see a serious federal commitment to HIV services. We are still experiencing a bias against people with AIDS. We are still seeing a bias against New York State and New York City as the epicenter of the epidemic. Some examples:

❑ This coming year, CDC funding to New York State's Bureau of Prevention will be at least $5 million short of what is needed merely to support the current contracts, to say nothing of meeting the need for vastly expanded prevention services.

❑ Although the New York-New Jersey area had more than 40 percent of the country's IV drug users with AIDS, the Health Resources and Services Administration (HRSA) decided not long ago to award the area only 8 percent of the money available for integrated primary care and substance-abuse services.

❒ New York State has about 30 percent of the reported pediatric AIDS cases. Yet HRSA awarded New York only $1.6 million—about 15 percent—of the $10.4 million available to fund new Pediatric AIDS Demonstration Projects.

New York has, in fact, done quite a lot on its own. Much of the state's leadership in the area of AIDS has come from the AIDS Institute, established as a result of the vision of former Health Commissioner David Axelrod and Governor Cuomo to address this unique plague. Together with other state agencies, the institute has implemented a broad and creative variety of programs. We should be proud of what it has been able to accomplish.

Nationally as well, the outlook for those with HIV infection, while still grim, has improved. Early detection is now encouraged by all since prophylactic care and medical treatment of symptomatic HIV infection prolong life and often prevent recurring hospitalizations. Earlier counseling and testing help to prevent the spread of infection to sexual partners. Discrimination, while still rampant, has lessened noticeably in some quarters.

These accomplishments are the result of national efforts by a vast array of medical, social, economic, educational, and legal experts. That is what AIDS demands. The epidemic of HIV infection is a *national* disaster. Its concentration in populous cities reflects its dependence on risk behavior and social factors that are more prevalent and more visible in cities. But AIDS is spreading slowly and surely to suburban and rural areas. States and local communities can do their share, and many have done as much as they possibly can without dismantling other critical programs and services. They cannot do it alone. They should not be expected to shoulder this devastating and unprecedented burden individually.

AIDS must be recognized not only as a national problem, but one that requires a heroic response outside of the standard public health allocations. Just as we should not disband the Coast Guard to pay for the Persian Gulf war, we cannot take money from lead poisoning or measles immunization programs to pay for AIDS.

The defeat of AIDS must not only be seen as a national priority, requiring an extraordinary national response, but as a battle that we can win. Unlike many other major killers, AIDS is completely preventable. Existing preventive education programs work. There are simply not enough of them.

What do we need? Quite a lot if we are to fulfill our public health mandate and behave like the responsible, compassionate people we wish to be. Clearly, we are in the midst of a fiscal crisis, but that is not an excuse to decide that decent public health care is expendable or that we can ignore the most urgent health crisis of our time. We are not poor; we are stingy. We must do what we clearly see is necessary, by reordering our national priorities and, if necessary, by taking on greater expenses ourselves.

We need a crisis team, crisis financing, and coordinated federal, state, and local leadership. We need strong medical and social-service infrastructures in community and health organizations. We need more primary care, personnel, housing, and home care. We need aggressive, explicit preventive education for children, adolescents, and adults.

We need to agree that these efforts are worth the price. We can, if we want, forestall the needless suffering and death inherent in all of our major public health crises, including AIDS. Our society and our health-care systems can afford to meet these challenges and our other health and social needs as well. Only by not doing so will we be truly impoverished.

The Economic Consequences of Inaction

❖ Marianne C. Fahs ❖

The tragic and threatening consequences of the fiscal epidemic of health-care cutbacks in the City of New York
illustrate in miniature the profound consequences that
lie ahead for the health of the nation as a whole. We are rapidly becoming a nation of big cities. Thirty years ago, less
than two-thirds of the country was urban. Today, over three-
fourths of our population is urban. One hundred of our 250
million live in the largest twenty metropolitan areas.[1] The challenges we face in New York are the challenges we face as an
urban nation, striving to maintain a competitive edge as
we look ahead to the twenty-first century.

For the past fifteen years, I have been studying the relationship
between economic productivity and illness. My research, and
that of others in this field, shows the economic consequences
of illness to our society to be vast. They include the direct medical costs of providing health care to the ill—the consequences most often cited in policy circles. But they also
include the incalculable toll in human pain and suffering that
disease costs American families and friends every year, and
the devastating costs to our economic viability as a city, and
as a nation, through significant losses in economic productivity due to disease.

The economic consequences of illness are staggering.[2] The
annual loss in productivity to our national economy associated
with work loss due to illness and premature death is now over
$450 billion. This represents over 10 percent of our total eco-
nomic production. Think of the tremendous boost to the
economy and to our competitive world position that would

result if we were able to harness this economic potential. The disturbing truth of the matter is that, according to standard preventive medicine textbooks, we *are* able to prevent over 90 percent of this economic productivity loss, using current knowledge and technology.

AIDS, "the most devastating epidemic of our century," adds an accelerating toll to our economic loss.[3] Published estimates indicate the loss in economic productivity associated with AIDS is especially high, because this disease strikes young people, often at the beginning of their most productive years. In 1991, the productive loss to our economy associated with AIDS is estimated to be over $55.6 billion.[4]

While this is a national problem, New York is especially hard hit, and shoulders a disproportionate share of this loss. With 21 percent of the nation's AIDS cases in New York State, AIDS costs the New York State economy over $12 billion annually; $10 billion of that loss is contributed by the toll this devastating epidemic takes in New York City.[5]

We are a nation of communities. But the real cutbacks in federal support of community health programs in the 1980s, combined with the absence of federal leadership in instituting comprehensive health-care reform, have resulted in a shift of responsibility to state and local governments. Cities and states have been left to fend for themselves. What constituted hard times in the 1980s, during a period of economic expansion, constitutes a real crisis in 1991. I do not use that term lightly. It is in fact both a fiscal and a moral crisis.

The 1980s was a period of economic expansion for some, but not for others. From 1979 to 1987, the standard of living of the top fifth of the population rose by 19 percent. At the same time, the living standard for the more than forty million Americans who make up the poorest fifth of the population fell by 9 percent.[6] According to the Census Bureau, the income gap between the richest and the poorest is now wider than it has been at any time since the bureau began keeping such statistics in 1947.

During the 1980s, the poor became both poorer and more numerous.[7] The percent of the American population living below the poverty line increased from 12.3 percent in 1975 to 13.1 percent in 1988. In New York State, the percent of Americans living below the poverty line increased from 6.7 to 8.7 percent; in New York City, from 15.0 percent to 20.8 percent. The annual rate of increase is accelerating.[8]

Particularly disturbing is the record regarding children. From 1975 to 1987, the poverty rate for children in the United States increased from 16 to 20 percent.[9] Today, one out of every five children in this country lives in poverty. This is more than double the rates found in Organization for Economic Cooperation and Development (OECD) countries.[10] In New York City, the poverty rate for children is double the national average; 40 percent of the city's children live in poverty. Fully 60 percent of the city's children live in families with incomes below 200 percent of the poverty level, compared with 43 percent nationally.[11]

There is a direct relationship between poverty and the prevalence of serious disease (see Figure below). To quote one

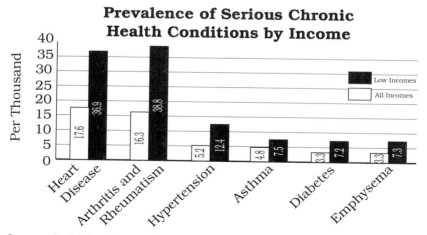

Prevalence of Serious Chronic Health Conditions by Income

Per Thousand

Low Incomes
All Incomes

Heart Disease: 17.6 / 36.9
Arthritis and Rheumatism: 16.3 / 38.8
Hypertension: 5.2 / 12.4
Asthma: 4.8 / 7.5
Diabetes: 3.3 / 7.2
Emphysema: 3.3 / 7.3

Source: R. J. Blendon and D. E. Rogers, "Cutting Medical Care Costs," *Journal of the American Medical Association*, vol. 250, no. 14, October 14, 1983, pp. 1880-85. Copyright 1983, American Medical Association.

of the great leaders in the history of public health, Johann Peter Frank, "poverty is the chief cause of disease."[12] The federal government found that the percentage of people in the United States who consider themselves in only fair or poor health (as opposed to good, very good, or excellent health) rises precipitously as income level drops: from 4.6 percent for people with incomes over $35,000 to 21.1 percent for people with incomes below $10,000. The number of bed disability days per year is three times as high for people with incomes under $5,000 as compared to people with incomes above $25,000.[13]

What does this increase in poverty and decline in health have to do with the nation's economy? Radical reductions of funding in public health have dire consequences beyond the crippling of our ability to meet the many health needs of Americans. The short-term saving in health expenditures is, in the long run, illusionary, as the following cases illustrate.

Thwarted Promises in Our Nation's Communities

❐ LEAD POISONING. Lead poisoning is the most common and socially devastating disease of young children, currently damaging the intelligence and behavior of at least 3 million to 4 million children in the United States (17 percent of all children).[14] Vulnerability to lead poisoning is associated with poverty. This invisible epidemic will cost the country over $28 billion during the next twenty years.[15]

Control of this epidemic will save the U.S. economy money. Research shows that a $34 billion investment in lead poisoning prevention programs over a twenty year period will *save* $62 billion in monetized returns, through averted health-care costs, increased income associated with increased IQ, and averted special-education costs.[16]

The tragedy we face today in cities such as New York is a drastic cut in lead poisoning prevention programs. The consequences of this loss of public health leadership and vision will inevitably be borne by all of us in the form of higher taxes and further losses in productivity, as we bear the double burden of increased medical and educational costs for our affected children, and as we find our economic GNP growing more slowly than it could have, due to the disability of these individuals. The true tragedy here is that a concerted effort could virtually eliminate this disease in this country within twenty years—at substantial savings to our economy. To quote Primo Levi, "When we know how to reduce the torment, but do not do it, then we become the tormentors."[17]

❐ PREVENTION OF LOW BIRTH WEIGHT. In the 1980s, after years of slow decline, there was an actual increase in the percentage of infants born with low birth weight, the most significant factor in determining infant death and disability.[18] The Office of Technology (OTA) estimates that for every low birth weight birth averted by earlier and more frequent prenatal care, the U.S. health-care system saves between $14,000 and $30,000 in newborn hospitalization, rehospitalizations in the first year, and long-term health-care costs associated with low birth weight.[19] The OTA reports that encouraging poor women to obtain early prenatal care through expanded public health benefits is a good investment for the nation. Further, the OTA underestimates the true savings to the economy: If the disabilities associated with low birth weight are averted, we can expect an increase in productivity.

Yet the percentage of women receiving early and regular prenatal care declined significantly in the 1980s. In 1987, more than 74,000 pregnant women received no prenatal care at all— a 50 percent increase over the 1980 rate.[20] Unfortunately, as a consequence of the proposed Fiscal Year 1992 budget cuts, all public maternity, education, and referral services would be eliminated in New York City. The 10,000 women who are currently being served by maternity and family planning services, and an estimated 18,300 newly enrolled clients in 1992, would not receive referrals to prenatal, postpartum, or well-child care.

❐ CHILDHOOD IMMUNIZATION. The cost-effectiveness of childhood vaccines is well established in the scientific literature.

The first twenty years of measles vaccination provided a net savings to the U.S. economy of $5.1 billion.[21] A 1983 study showed that the use of a combined measles, mumps, and rubella vaccine saved the country $60 million in direct medical costs and increased productivity.[22] Another study, in 1984, of pertussis vaccination showed a $44 million savings in medical costs for every one million children vaccinated.[23]

Despite the clearly established economic benefits, the current levels of immunization in this country are less than half of those in the United Kingdom, France, Canada, Israel, Spain, Italy, and Sweden.[24] And Dr. James Mason, head of the U.S. Public Health Service, points out: "The current outbreak of measles is an ominous foreshadowing of what could be in store, if we don't make rapid progress in raising immunization coverage of preschoolers. . . . We could be laying the foundation for outbreaks of diphtheria, pertussis, polio, mumps, rubella, and congenital rubella syndrome."[25]

With the increase in poverty among our nation's children, and the real cutbacks in health and income-support programs of the early 1980s, preventable childhood diseases are on the rise. Unfortunately, as a consequence of the proposed Fiscal Year 1992 budget cuts, over 100,000 immunizations given annually at walk-in immunization clinics in New York City would be eliminated.

□ CERVICAL CANCER AND LOW-INCOME ELDERLY WOMEN. A study conducted by the Department of Community Medicine at Mount Sinai of a cervical cancer screening program for elderly women attending a municipal hospital outpatient clinic in New York City showed that for every one hundred Pap smears performed, the screening program saved the health-care system over $5,000. Odd as it may seem, this study, published only three years ago, was the first economic analysis in this country of public health prevention efforts among the low-income elderly.[26] Unfortunately, the $5.4 million proposed cut in laboratory services run by the Department of Health would simply eliminate Pap smear testing from its laboratory services program.

These four examples lay bare some of the economic impli-
cations of the public health disaster we are facing in the
communities of our nation. We are mortgaging our future by
systematically destroying our human and economic potential. Further, with the increased suffering we are imposing
on our poor, we are becoming a morally bankrupt society.

How did we arrive at such a predicament? It is not as though
we haven't been trying to solve the interrelated and complex
problems of health, productivity, and economic growth for
some time. In the past few years, we have seen the arrival
of one reform after another—all with little success. We must
find new strength in the face of adversity, for the serious problems facing us are soluble. As Winston Churchill said:
"Americans can always be relied on to do the right thing after
they have exhausted all the other possibilities."

The Myths about the Health-Care Cost Crisis

The United States, which spends 12 percent of its GNP on
health care (a percentage that has been steadily increasing
over time), has higher expenditures for health care than any
other nation.[27] This statistic usually accompanies the hand-
wringing over our current "health-care cost crisis." Since the
late 1970s, the policy response to this "crisis" has increasingly
focused on reducing government expenditure on health
care. The assumption is that health-care expenditure increases should be fought by ever more draconian cuts to our
public health-care budgets. This is wrong-headed policy.
Health-care expenditures are not full economic costs, and, as
the above examples show, cuts in government health expenditures can actually increase the full economic costs we bear.

After fifteen years of health-care reform failures under
Presidents Carter, Reagan, and Bush, who have all tried to
follow traditional economic principles of competition and allow
the "invisible hand" of the market to rule the production and
distribution of health in the United States, the American

public is ready for a major change. Poll after poll demonstrates that there is a crisis of confidence in the American health-care system.[28] Yet today's policy responses continue to be based on economic myths that lack supporting empirical evidence.

❏ MYTH #1: CUTS IN HEALTH-CARE EXPENDITURES ELIMINATE HEALTH-CARE SERVICES ONLY. There is a fundamental principle in economics, that expenditures equal income. Health care in fact, because it is labor intensive, creates a high rate of jobs per expenditure—much higher than, say, military expenditures, which are capital intensive. Today, health care employs thirty-seven out of every one thousand Americans, compared with twenty-eight out of every one thousand ten years ago.[29] The number of health-related employees surged from 6.1 million in 1979 to 8.7 million in 1989—by 43 percent. According to Labor and Census Department estimates, by the end of the 1990s, at least twelve million Americans will work in health services, which will contain seven of the ten fastest growing occupations.[30] Cuts in public health budgets not only deny people needed medical care, they also deny people jobs.

❏ MYTH #2: HEALTH-CARE SPENDING BY BUSINESS DESTROYS AMERICA'S COMPETITIVENESS. It is an unproved myth that health-care spending adversely affects America's "competitiveness."[31] According to this widely shared folklore, an automobile produced in Detroit now contains between $500 and $700 of health-care costs. But as Uwe Reinhardt, professor of economics at Princeton University, argues, it is not high health-care costs *per se*—in the form of insurance premiums and fringe benefits—that render American business non-competitive at home or abroad, it is the *total* worker-compensation package—benefits *plus* cash wages—that affects business competitiveness.[32] In fact, workers have accepted trade-offs of cash income for fringe benefits, so that total compensation packages remain competitive.[33]

❏ MYTH #3: HEALTH-CARE SPENDING BY THE GENERAL PUBLIC DESTROYS AMERICA'S COMPETITIVENESS. It is highly unlikely that

the relatively large percentage of the American GNP devoted to health care, by itself, adversely affects the nation's
competitiveness. Economists are quick to point out that
there is nothing magical about the current percentage of
our economy spent on health care.[34] Not only is it not necessarily wrong to spend 12 percent of our economic wealth
on health care, but we could even spend substantially more—
say 20 percent—without adversely affecting other productive sectors of the economy.

In 1987, Americans spent a total of $194 billion on hospi-
tal care, $102 billion on physician services, and $34 billion on
drugs and sundries. While these are sizable outlays, that same
year Americans spent $35.6 billion on tobacco, $61 billion on
alcohol, $24.2 billion on jewelry, and $26.2 billion on cosmetics.[35]
Arguments that spending in health care is a misallocation of
productive resources must contend with these statistics.

❏ MYTH #4: HEALTH-CARE SPENDING BY THE GOVERNMENT
DESTROYS AMERICA'S COMPETITIVENESS. The only way in which
high health expenditures are likely to detract from the
nation's competitiveness in the long run is if public health-
care spending comes at the expense of our investment in other
forms of human capital (such as education) or the nation's
infrastructure, both of which are largely publicly financed.[36]
And this would only happen if the American taxpayers and
their political representatives insist on keeping the percentage of GNP going through public budgets constant—so that
more spent on public health care (about 41 percent of all health
expenditures at the present time) means less spent on other
public programs.[37]

Our tax burden in this country (33 percent of the GNP)
remains lower than that of all the European nations in OECD,
where tax-to-GNP ratios range in the mid-to-high 40 percent
range.[38] We maintain the lowest tax burden despite a growing underclass of poverty-stricken children, an increase in the
elderly population, and higher infant mortality rates and lower
life expectancies than in almost all other OECD countries.[39]

Research shows a strong positive correlation between public health expenditures as a percent of GNP and life expectancy.[40] Countries that place a high priority on health programs have approximately two to three times lower infant mortality and child death rates than their counterparts at the same level of economic development.[41]

Further, the United States has the lowest public health to total health expenditure ratio of all twenty-four OECD countries; at 41 percent it is comparable only to Turkey.[42] Other countries average between 70 and 80 percent. This higher public health allocation does not adversely affect their GNP growth. For example, in comparison with Canada and Japan, our average annual GNP growth per capita between 1985 and 1988 in real dollars ranks a poor third.[43]

In New York City, the public health-care budget did not keep pace with the growth in real GNP during the 1980s, and it has been continually losing ground in real dollars. But the substantial restrictions of the proposed 1992 budget mark the first reversal in public health expenditures. There is no doubt that the impact of these shrinking resources will adversely affect the city's health. Econometric analyses have shown a quantifiable direct relationship between health expenditures and age-adjusted mortality.[44] Based on these equations, we can expect our age-adjusted mortality in New York to increase.

The Legacy of Laissez-Faire

Current federal inaction is based on the economic theory of competition, which embodies the principle of *laissez-faire*—literally, let the private market alone to do its work. The Reagan and Bush administrations have used the theoretical ideal of competition and "privatization" to sound the alarm against rising public health-care expenditures. This alarm is combined illogically with the reassurance that public program cuts and stiffer hospital and physician regulation will solve the cost problem.

Competition used this way is a wolf in sheep's clothing. The theory, as first detailed by Adam Smith in his classic *The Wealth of Nations*, predicts that the ultimate outcome of the God-like "invisible hand" guiding the private market will be compatible with both private profitseeking and the public benefit. But even Adam Smith had moral qualms about this compatibility. According to Smith, the interest of those who live by profit "is never exactly the same as that of the public," and they "have generally an interest to deceive and even to oppress the public, and . . . accordingly have, upon many occasions, both deceived and oppressed it."[45]

Moral qualms aside, the economic and health policy literature is full of reasoned arguments and empirical proof that the special quality of health care does not meet the stringent requirements necessary before the ideals of competition can be approached.[46] For example, consumers must have time to search the market to exercise their sovereignty, yet medical care requirements are often urgent, leaving no time to shop for the best price. There must be free entry into the market, which goes absolutely against the standards of the AMA and state licensor boards. And consumers must have perfect knowledge about the quality of the product, which is extremely difficult to attain in the complex and constantly changing field of medicine.

The past decade of "competition" in health care has brought four adverse consequences:

❑ CONSEQUENCE #1: HIGHER COSTS. National health-care spending has more than doubled from $248 billion in 1980 to over $600 billion this year—a spending increase of $1,000 per person. Adjusted for inflation, health-care expenditures have been growing at near record levels.[47]

❑ CONSEQUENCE #2: INCREASED REGULATION. The "market"-oriented policies of the Reagan and Bush administrations have left us with an erosion of clinical freedom. Physicians in the United States are now the most litigated-against, second-guessed, and paperwork-laden physicians in Western industrialized democracies. Rates of malpractice suits against private-practice physicians more than tripled between 1980 and 1985.[48]

❒ CONSEQUENCE #3: LOSS OF HEALTH INSURANCE FOR AMERICANS WHO NEED IT MOST. Because of the rising cost of health insurance premiums, insurance companies, including even Blue Cross, have responded to competition by dropping "bad risks." The horrible irony is that these are the people who need coverage most. The numbers of uninsured have increased from 30 million in 1980 to approximately 37 million in 1987, and millions more are underinsured.[49]

Further, the proportion of children in the United States without private or public health insurance increased from about 13 percent in 1977 to 18 percent in 1987.[50] Today, one-third of all poor and low-income children have no health insurance. This is a consequence of the decrease in private coverage among low-income families, and the decrease in public coverage of single-parent families.[51] Again, the tragedy is that these are children with the highest health needs; among the poor and near-poor, there is an increased incidence of respiratory infections, tuberculosis, measles, dysentery, childhood lead poisoning, and AIDS.

❒ CONSEQUENCE #4: DETERIORATING ADMINISTRATIVE EFFICIENCY. Because many different health insurance companies compete with each other in the United States, the proportion of health-care expenditures consumed by administration—in the form of insurance overhead, hospital administration, nursing home administration, and physicians' overhead and billing expenses—is higher than in Canada and in Britain, where there is a single-payer system. In 1983, administrative costs in the United States were 60 percent higher than in Canada and 97 percent higher than in Britain.[52] Further, between 1983 and 1987, administrative costs in the United States increased 37 percent in real dollars, whereas in Canada they declined. The proportion of health-care spending consumed by administration is now at least 117 percent higher in the United States than in Canada.[53]

Options for the Future

The economic consequences of public health inaction are severe. They include direct health expenditures, due to the costs of disease that could have been prevented, and decreases in worker productivity potential. It is an economic truism that investment in capital increases labor productivity. Our neglect of *human* capital investment will surely decrease our rate of GNP increase; health is a crucial contributor to economic growth.

Health-care spending is a productive use of resources. We must educate the American public to understand what a payoff the right kind of public spending can have. If we lose the productivity of our poor and near poor, we lose a profound American dream—the dream of betterment, of the poor or working-class immigrants who work hard so that their children can go to college. The evidence is clear that the loss of access to health care during the 1980s is already robbing many Americans and their children of an opportunity for a long, healthy, and productive life. A young *uninsured* adult male now has three times the chance of dying during a hospitalization as an *insured* adult male, similar in every way except for insurance status.[54] The death of such a man can mean the end of the American dream for his young children, who must attempt the struggle toward economic improvement without the financial support of their father; it is a preventable tragedy.

In order to achieve the economic expansion we are capable of, we must adopt an active public health policy agenda, with target objectives *and* target budgets clearly spelled out. Without a federal economic and political agenda for the health of the nation, we are in danger of lurching off track each time political pressures present unexpected choices.

Our economic growth depends on our public health investments of today. Government can simply look the other way or can summon the courage to face the problem squarely.

A good investment choice is to reduce the number of Americans living in poverty. One way to approach this problem efficiently, without increasing taxes, is to decrease income disparity through a negative income tax policy. This policy would redistribute the tax burden more equitably among income brackets, with the lowest brackets getting cash returns.

Another investment choice is to form a federal community partnership to improve access to health care. The decrease in funding to community health centers has had a devastating impact on the poor served by these programs. This has been a myopic cost-cutting policy. These programs are a cost-effective use of federal health expenditures; they are targeted on high-need populations; and they have been highly successful in reducing the hospitalization rates—from 25 percent to 67 percent—of those served.[55]

How could this partnership be financed? One way is to make sure that all community health center clients are already insured when they arrive at the health center. We have the capability to achieve that at the present time, with no additional taxes. The General Accounting Office reports that *if the United States went to a single-payer system of paying for medical care*, similar to that in Canada, *the annual savings would be $75 billion*. This is more than enough to cover all the uninsured, with enough left over to cover all the deductibles, copayments and out-of-pocket costs for medical care to all others presently insured.[56] This reform offers President Bush a historic opportunity to guarantee basic health care to every American.

But to rebuild our public health infrastructure and increase the availability and accessibility of health services to our disadvantaged communities, we need both new, creative, and culturally sensitive community programs and outreach efforts, as well as new investment capital for these efforts. We can have higher taxes, or we can have *different* taxes. We might consider reviewing federal excise taxes on alcohol and cigarettes, which have been very stable since 1951.[57] Research by Michael Grossman, professor of economics at the City University of New York, shows that if we were to raise the excise tax on beer in line with the rate of inflation over the past three decades, we would cut motor-vehicle fatalities of eighteen to twenty-year-olds (many of which are alcohol related) by about 15 percent, saving more than one thousand lives per year. If we were to restore the excise tax on cigarettes to its real value in 1951, 800,000 premature deaths of Americans twelve years and older would be averted.[58] These can be considered public health investment taxes. If they are used to improve services to the poor, they will have a public health multiplier effect on both national health levels and economic wealth.

We remain a nation of communities. Some of our communities are desperately ill. We cannot ignore them. The cost is too high. We must fight against ignorance, political expediency, and selfishness to uphold the ideals of community medicine, first advanced a generation ago by Dr. Kurt Deuschle, the founder of community medicine in the United States. As he has said, "In the final analysis, the diagnosis and treatment of community and social pathology, not individual pathology, must be our major concern."[59]

Our public health programs are among the most cost-effective health programs in the country. Action must come soon or health-care problems will bring this country to its knees. The most rapid and dramatic improvements in the health of the public will result not from technology-intensive medical care but from preventive measures. These are grossly underfunded at the present time; only 2.9 percent of all health dollars is spent for government public health activities. We must turn away from the narrow-minded cost-containment refrains to consider the health of our country. We need rational analysis, compassion, and an appreciation of the long-run, as well as the sort-run, aspects of this complex problem.

As Joseph Califano, former secretary of the Department of Health, Education and Welfare, wrote in his autobiography:

"Of course, those who govern will make mistakes. Plenty of them. But we should not fear failure. What we should fear above all is the judgment of God and the judgment of history if we, the most affluent people on earth, free to choose and act as we wish, choose not to govern justly, choose not to distribute our riches fairly and to help the most vulnerable among us, or worse yet, choose not to even try."

The Private Sector: Good Partners in Hard Times

❖ *James Jones and Deborah Steelman, Esq.* ❖

It has long been an axiom that more is accomplished through cooperation than through decree. Nowhere is that axiom more applicable than in health-care reform. Cooperation embodied in a public/private partnership is needed for three principal reasons:

1. the upcoming challenges for health-care financing are too great and the problems too complex for one sector to address alone;
2. the public and private sectors each have advantages that are instrumental in addressing any viable solution; and
3. cooperation is essential for building consensus, and consensus is essential for reform.

As this nation prepares for the challenges of the twenty-first century, this partnership will play an especially important role in reform of the public health system.

Challenges of the Future

Today's health-care reform debate contains two principal focal points:

1. the problem of access to health care for the 15 percent of our population without health-care coverage, and
2. the dizzying spiral of growing health-care costs.

The access to health-care issue is overwhelmed by the health-care cost-growth problem. In terms of the health-care reform debate, an appropriate analogy for the access/cost issue might be that the people in the house are complaining that the plumbing is not working when the whole house is beginning to burn. Both problems need attention. The issue is the order in which they are addressed.

Health-care costs are and have been increasing for well over three decades. Health-care expenditures today are consuming more than 12 percent of gross national product (GNP)—more than in any other nation. Americans spend nearly $700 billion a year on health care, and this amount is expected to increase at a dramatic rate. Unpublished preliminary estimates—estimates that use somewhat optimistic assumptions—project health care to consume about 31.5 percent of GNP in the year 2020. National health expenditures are projected to be close to $9.5 trillion in that year—nearly twice the entire GNP in the United States today. Further, these estimates simply project current law into the future—they assume no new programs or program changes.

Why is growth so high? It is often very tempting to pick one cause for one effect, but the factors contributing to the escalation in health-care costs are complex. One irreversible reason is that our society is aging. In 1990, there were thirty-two million Americans over the age of sixty-five. In 2020, that number is expected to be fifty-three million. The portion of the population over the age of sixty-five will go from 12 percent today to over 17 percent in the year 2020, and the portion over age eighty-five will double.

Although demographics contribute to escalating health-care costs, they are not the major factor. Many people believe that escalating health-care costs are primarily a result of the aging of the population, since older people consume more health-care dollars per capita. A panel of experts, which was convened by the 1991 Advisory Council on Social Security and is comprised of some of the nation's leading economists and actuaries, attempted to identify the amount of increasing health-care costs that were simply due to demographic changes—that is, the aging of the population.

Preliminary estimates indicate that no more than 10 percent of the predicted increase in health care's share of GNP is directly attributable to the aging of the population.

Also contributing to the burgeoning share of the GNP that health-care expenditures consume is the fact that our economy is not growing as fast as health-care costs are growing. Over the past ten years, real wages, a rough proxy for growth in per capita GNP, have grown about 0.8 percent annually. Using rather optimistic assumptions, real wages are projected to increase by 1.1 percent per year in the future. Real health-care expenditures, on the other hand, have increased over the past decade at the rate of 3.7 percent per year. Real health-care expenditures are expected to increase by 4.3 percent over the next ten years and 3.5 percent per year thereafter.

Macro-Economic Findings

The United States is not alone in having to deal with an aging population; other industrialized countries are facing the aging of their populations earlier than the United States. Current Japanese and German populations have aged almost to the same level the United States will reach in the year 2020. But the United States may not be as well equipped to address the problems of this aging population, as evidenced by our lower savings rate and the greater indebtedness of individuals, corporations, and government.

Moreover, the actions taken by other nations to address their own challenges may reduce the resource capacity of the United States to accommodate its own expanding elderly population. As a nation's population ages, it faces a larger population of elderly who are no longer active in the work force. That nation's workers must either produce the goods and services for the nonworking sector to consume, or must look for other ways to finance that consumption—such as selling off its foreign holdings. For example, Japan could divest itself of its significant holdings in U.S. real estate and debt to pay for its elderly's consumption.

While other nations have been investing heavily in the United States for the past several years, the United States has not been investing as heavily abroad. This means that while other countries may choose to sell the assets they hold here, the United States cannot divest as rapidly abroad, and our balance of trade problems will be exacerbated. The flow of capital from our nation to other nations means fewer resources for our own consumption—that is, fewer resources to pay for health care, education, and so forth.

Another aspect of the issue of the aging of our population relates to the future costs of our social insurance programs, to which most of our elderly will be entitled. In the year 2020, the cost of Social Security and Medicare is projected to be equivalent to about 25 percent of taxable payroll. That means that one-fourth of all the wages and self-employment that are subject to the Social Security payroll tax will go toward sustaining these two programs for the elderly—and that does not include long-term care.

Can the United States sustain this growth in health-care expenditures? It became very clear to the panel that we as a nation cannot continue to have the consumption patterns we enjoy today and accommodate such growth in health-care expenditures. In fact, for these patterns to continue, preliminary estimates indicate that the GNP would have to be 32 percent greater than what government actuaries project that it will be, even with somewhat optimistic assumptions in real wage growth. Real wage growth would have to be nearly double what is currently projected. This means having real wage growth of 2.2 percent per year in order to accommodate the increasing share that health care will consume—a wage growth not seen in this country since the 1950s.

Judging from the average real wage growth rate in the United States over the past ten years, this is a problem Americans probably will not be able to "outgrow." In fact, the projected medical expenditures will grow so much that, unless other consumption is substantially curtailed, investment will become negative, leading to steadily declining real income. Americans will all have less to spend on goods and services. But even more importantly, negative investment would severely curtail the nation's ability to produce goods and services competitively in a world market.

Micro-Economic Findings

Just as nations may be faced with divesting assets to pay for the retirement of their respective baby boomers, so will individuals be seeking ways to divest to pay for consumption in their retirements. Those fifty-three million Americans over age sixty-five in the year 2020 may very well be selling their assets—primarily their homes—to finance their retirements. And, as discussed earlier, the divestiture of foreign countries already will have been driving real estate prices down. In addition, due to changing demographics, there will be fewer buyers, bringing prices down further. America's baby boomers will be faced with paying high prices for their homes in their working years, but receiving lower prices when they attempt to sell those homes to help pay for their retirements. In other words, baby boomers will have bought high and sold low.

Further, at the same time society will be faced with paying the increased costs of Social Security and Medicare for baby boomers, these retirees will be faced with increasing Medicare premiums. The average retiree in 2020 is projected to pay a Medicare Part B premium that consumes 13.3 percent of his or her Social Security benefit. Other Medicare cost-sharing could bring this up to around 50 percent of his or her monthly check.

This challenging picture underscores a point made at the beginning: *If health-care expenditures increase at the projected rate, it will be too enormous a burden for either the public or private sector to finance alone.* The federal, state, and local governments' budgets are already strained today. It is doubtful that they will be any less strained in 2020. Furthermore, it is doubtful that the private sector of 2020 could come up with the necessary financing on its own. Americans have done about all they can to maintain real family income in the face of sluggish growth in productivity and real wages per worker. They have had fewer children, sent more household members into the labor market, and kept savings low and debt levels high—all of which in the past have helped stretch incomes to cover expenses. It seems likely, however, that trends in making ends meet by having fewer children, saving less, or borrowing more, and having two-earner families are reaching their limits. Yet reconciling high expectations with limited resources will be difficult in light of the expected political pressure from a voting elderly population that will be nearly double what it is today. Our capacity from these strategies is nearly depleted; new strategies are needed.

Improving Public Health:
Part of the Solution

One strategy to address this problem would be to find a method of increasing productivity. Historically, large increases in productivity have been associated with advances in cost-reducing technology resulting from research and development. For example, developments in agricultural technology have allowed units of food to be produced with fewer farmers and other workers. This has lowered costs and has been translated into higher productivity and, eventually, into higher GNP.

In health care, however, although research and development has led to technological advances in diagnosing diseases and in prolonging life, these technological advances have resulted in an increase in the number of health-care personnel to run the costly machinery. This has resulted in higher unit costs and, therefore, lower productivity. Some argue that this is only true because technology such as Magnetic Resonance Imaging (MRI) is underutilized, and therefore is inefficient. But use of additional personnel occurs even when the technology is operated with maximum efficiency. This is because much of the new technology is more labor intensive as well as more expensive to use. A prominent economist likened the development of health-care technology to that of movie and theater technology. The quality of the pictures, sound, special effects, and comfort of the theaters have improved, but technology has done nothing to reduce the costs of seeing a movie.

Cost-reducing technologies are needed to deal with health-expenditure growth. Cost-reducing technologies are not limited to machines; they include methods of combining resources that are effective, efficient, and productive. Examples of health-care delivery that have possessed many of those attributes, and can contribute to solving the health-cost problem, can be found in the public health system.

But, as it stands today, the infrastructure of the American public health system is not adequately prepared to deal with many of the health problems of today and of the future. Over the past several decades, the United States has seen a decline in the foundation of its public health system. Public hospitals are bearing a tremendous burden in caring for those who have no other source of health care and do not have sufficient capacity to do so. Patients who visit emergency rooms or ambulatory screening clinics may spend up to twenty hours navigating their way through the system—including triage at the emergency room, waiting to be seen by a doctor or nurse, having lab tests done, and waiting for their prescriptions to be filled. Emergency room patients often lie on beds in crowded hallways because there is either no doctor to see them or no hospital bed available. An August 1991 *JAMA* article reported on patients leaving emergency rooms unseen after hours of waiting.

Our cities are deluged by the results of crack cocaine and other addictions. Initial treatment for a baby delivered to a crack-cocaine-addicted mother can easily cost $150,000 to $200,000. These babies then become boarder babies at six or seven months old, and, unwanted, they may be discharged directly to a homeless shelter or become wards of the state or city. No one knows what the future will be for these children—the long-range effects of crack cocaine addiction from birth are just becoming known—and it does not look good for the already taxed American school systems. Patterns of sudden, erratic, violent, and abusive behavior are beginning to emerge—along with long-term intellectual impairment and other development disabilities. Americans will pay an increasing cost for this disease.

In the 1950s and 1960s, specialized public hospitals dealt with epidemic diseases, such as tuberculosis and polio. The public health system was economically efficient. As these diseases were eradicated, the beds that were available for treatment were closed, health-care manpower was redeployed, and efforts of private foundations, such as the March of Dimes and Christmas Seals, were redirected.

The present structural foundation of the public health system is simply insufficient to handle the massive health problems the United States is facing. For example, philosophical changes, new approaches to treatment, court cases, and a rash of publicity caused a shift in the treatment of mental illness from inpatient to outpatient—and resulted in a decline in inpatient and residential treatment facilities by more than 50 percent from 1970 through 1982. State and county public facilities, which account for more than 44 percent of all such facilities, declined from 413,000 to 199,000 between the years 1970 and 1986. One unfortunate by-product of this has been that one-third of all homeless are chronically mentally ill patients—many of whom were formerly cared for in hospitals.

The public health support in primary care has also suffered. As school enrollment declined after the baby boomers passed through school systems, cuts to school budgets forced the elimination of school nurses and school clinics. Neighborhood health centers and well-baby clinics, which flourished in the 1960s and 1970s, declined sharply during the late 1970s and 1980s. Shifts in family structure—that is from one-earner families to two-earner families, coupled with a rise in single, working parents—have resulted in a need for services for the children of baby boomers. The percentage of young children who are fully immunized against childhood infectious diseases has been decreasing steadily; measles, thought to be eradicated in the early 1980s, has reappeared in epidemic form—a twelvefold increase in just seven years. Tuberculosis and sexually transmitted diseases, such as syphilis and hepatitis, are also on the rise.

The United States needs to strengthen its public health system—a system that in the past not only provided public health education and disease prevention, but also, in troubled times, the health care for those without. Strengthening the public health system is not only morally and ethically the right thing to do, it is the smart thing to do. In the light of changing demographics—a predicted decline in the number of active workers per retiree—it makes good sense, good economic sense, to ensure that the nation has healthy, bright children growing up in healthy environments to become a solid and productive work force for the future.

The strengthening of the public health infrastructure in the United States is achievable and necessary, regardless of the outcome of the debate on health-care financing. An insurance card is not of much help to a crack-addicted mother, and certainly will not prevent AIDS, or even ensure that pre-school-aged children receive the immunizations and other medical care that they need. Health insurance does not coordinate the educational, social, transportation, and health services often needed to address the problem. Public health programs, clinics, and centers—both privately or publicly financed or run—have traditionally done so, and generally have done well. We believe that the focus on the access issue should be switched from access to insurance coverage to access to health care. When one does that, the potential strengths of improving the public health system become evident.

Public/Private Partnership

To rehabilitate the public health infrastructure, and prepare for tomorrow, the nation must capitalize on the different strengths of the public and private sectors. It has worked successfully in the past, and the size and complexity of future problems necessitates even greater reliance on the different strengths that each sector can bring to bear.

The public sector plays an important role. It provides an overall structure and direction to public health activities by establishing policies, standards, and goals:

❑ The federal government stimulates discussion and debate on issues related to the public health. Many state and city governments have recently created task forces of public officials and a wide range of interested organizations and individuals to assess what is needed in their communities to improve access to health services.

❑ The public sector plays an important role by coordinating a broad array of government-run services relating to food, housing, and transportation—areas obviously essential for good health.

❑ The federal government conducts a variety of important educational and informational activities. The Centers for Disease Control conducts national surveillance of communicable diseases, such as AIDS, and provides educational materials to state and local governments, health-care providers, and the public. The Agency for Health Care Policy and Research collects and disseminates statistics on the use of health-care services, and supports research or effective health-care treatment.

❑ The federal government plays a critical role marshalling significant financial resources to states, through block grants, to pay for and provide services.

❑ Federal and state governments provide care to millions of needy individuals in public hospitals and community and migrant health centers. Through the National Health Service Corps, physicians and other health professionals who received student loans to fund their medical educations receive loan forgiveness for providing health-care services in medically under-served rural and urban areas.

No one can dispute the important role the public sector plays in the area of public health, but, at times, the public sector can be inflexible. This can result in unintended harmful effects on the public health infrastructure.

For example, in Cuba, New Mexico, the ambulance service in town served an area of over 7,800 square miles—in a county that did not have a single hospital. The health clin-ic that operated this ambulance service did so to provide acute hospital care to its patients by transporting them to one of several hospitals in other counties. Because of budget con-straints, the clinic was faced with shutting down the ambu-lance service. It applied for, and received, a grant to keep the service operating—that is, until the granting agency found out that patients were being transported out of the county. The agency revoked the grant because rules and regula-tions dictated that funds could only be used for services performed within the borders of a single county. As a result of inflexible regulations, a community without a hospital lost an important source of support for its ambulance service.

This inflexibility underscores one of the strengths of the pri-vate sector. The private sector's flexibility comes from the fact that it has fewer constraints than the public sector, allowing for innovation that enables it to rapidly identify and fill gaps, target special groups and situations, and respond quickly to crises.

The capacity of the private sector to identify emerging needs and respond quickly was demonstrated when the AIDS epidemic developed. The disease became politicized in several communities and in some cases paralyzed the public sector's ability to provide a quick and timely response.

Private groups, however, demonstrated the capability and capacity to step in and raise money for research, counseling, treatment, and hospice care. Movie stars and other celebrities became actively involved in fund raising. Private clinics responded by shifting resources to produce services tailored to the HIV-infected. No matter what health reform emerges, we will always need this kind of capacity to rapidly respond to the next "AIDS-type" crises.

Privately donated services often fill critical gaps. More than one million Americans volunteer their services in the health-care field in any one year. For example, the Judeo-Christian Clinic in Florida relies solely on the services of over four hundred volunteer physicians, nurses, and other health-care professionals, who treat more than ten thousand patients free of charge. The clinic receives no government funds, and operates solely on donations. Guidelines for the clinic provide that those working poor not eligible for federal, state, and county health services programs will receive health care for free; patients are screened by a social worker or lay volunteers to determine financial eligibility. It is difficult to imagine a future in which no gaps in service will exist. The capacity of the private sector to respond to these gaps will continue to be relied upon.

Private foundations also play an important role in supporting new research and development. For example, the Robert Wood Johnson Foundation supports a wide variety of projects designed to demonstrate new models of efficient health-care service delivery in such areas as: outpatient health and supportive services for AIDS patients; primary care for underserved groups; community, day, and respite programs for those suffering with Alzheimer's disease; activities to support community efforts to reduce alcohol and drug abuse; and maternal and child health services.

The flexibility and innovation of these and other private-sector initiatives can contribute to a partnership with the public sector in financing, research and development, and delivery of public health services.

For example, the city of Albuquerque, New Mexico, in conjunction with the University of New Mexico, maintains school-based clinics in local elementary and senior high schools. A private computer company enabled this initiative to get off the ground by donating supplies and equipment—which were not available through public-funding means—to those clinics. The city provided the clinic, the university provided the physicians, and industry provided assistance tailored specifically to meet the immediate needs of the community. In 1990, corporations provided nearly $6 billion in philanthropic contributions of this kind.

Private/public partnerships have been particularly effective in public health research and development. Historically, the federal government, particularly the National Institutes of Health (NIH), has funded and conducted basic biomedical research into disease prevention. The private sector has applied these research findings to the development of vaccines and specific treatment regimens. This type of collaboration is reaching new dimensions in genome research. The public sector (NIH) offers ready access to some of the top scientists in the field, the infrastructure and patients for clinical trials, and the prestige associated with NIH activities; the private sector offers the flexibility to translate government science into health technology that may revolutionize treatment of disease.

Other examples of successful private/public partnerships include an outreach program for pregnant women living in city housing projects in Chicago. The local United Way agency, in conjunction with the city, operates this program, in which United Way employees work in project buildings and counsel women on prenatal care and appropriate care for their children once they are born. Another voluntary agency, the Red Cross, exemplifies public/private sector cooperation. This agency operates, among other things, our national blood banking system, provides immediate emergency disaster relief, and offers public health education and safety classes.

Conclusion

The public health system infrastructure is as important to our goals for economic growth and competitiveness as the physical infrastructure of the nation. Just as the nation needs good roads, water, and transportation systems to get products to market efficiently, the nation needs healthy workers to develop and produce those products competitively. It is incumbent on private-sector companies, foundations, and institutions to continue to be good partners—especially in hard times—by offering pharmaceuticals, machinery, supplies, and health-care providers on a pro bono basis. Creating the incentives and delivery framework to encourage private-sector participation must be a very high priority for both the president and Congress.

The days of the iron lung are long past, but the need to strengthen, reinforce, and, in places, restore the public health infrastructure to effectively and efficiently meet the public health problem is here today. The effort is too big for one sector alone. Only when the cooperative spirits of both the public and private sectors are re-energized will the nation be able to successfully solve this critical problem.

Part III:

New Approaches

Public health has had its legendary leaders, visionaries who prepared a better future by dealing with current disasters. In the midst of collapse, they devised better methods for controlling epidemics, and planted the seeds for a safer and healthier society.

In this section, Dr. Stephen B. Thacker proposes adapting the tools and lessons of modern warfare to meet the current challenges of public health. Congressman Charles Rangel, a senior member of the powerful Ways and Means Committee, represents one of the most impoverished communities in the country; he knows better than most how inadequate is the federal commitment to public health, and he speaks, more courageously than almost any of his colleagues, for the needs of the disenfranchised in American society. Mayor David N. Dinkins offers his analysis of the current healthcare crisis in New York, detailing the difficult decisions he made during a crippling fiscal crisis.

Finally, we have included the unedited transcript of Governor Mario M. Cuomo's presentation at the symposium that led to this volume. In a remarkable extemporaneous style, the governor offers an impassioned plea for a new set of national priorities to promote a domestic program of health and welfare that would try, once again, to fulfill the dreams of our Founding Fathers.

A War Room for Health

❖ Stephen B. Thacker, M.D. ❖

I want to introduce a concept called "Data for Decision Making." It is a concept of data-driven planning for health care, and it can be used to improve the budgeting process and to respond to health needs more efficiently in an era of diminishing resources. I believe it can be used successfully to address the problems of public health in the City of New York.

In health (and elsewhere), channels of communication between decisionmakers and technical experts are essential. Health information systems provide the indispensable quantitative basis. Technical experts gather and analyze the data, and then present findings and recommendations to the decisionmaker, who uses the data to articulate problems and goals and, ultimately, to formulate policies and programs that lead to action.

In this theoretical scenario, several assumptions are made about the process: that relevant data will be available and that this data will be recognized, appreciated, and utilized appropriately in the context of the existing social and cultural milieu. At the same time, we must assume that the technical experts will understand the problems articulated by decisionmakers, and that they can identify essential information, analyze data appropriately, and communicate information clearly and in a timely manner. Further, we must also assume that health information systems are operational and can provide accurate and timely data to the technical experts. Finally, we must assume that communications channels are effective, efficient, and sufficiently flexible to adapt to the changing needs of the health-care system. In theory, given these assumptions, policymakers can make rational and effective decisions. In practice, we know that in most situations, including in New York City, most of these assumptions are, at best, only partially true.

To address the gap between theory and practice, the Centers for Disease Control (CDC), in collaboration with the U.S. Agency for International Development, recently undertook a project to improve the decision-making process in health. We began this project with a series of case studies in Africa, Asia, and Latin America. The lessons learned are instructive.

In the 1980s, the emerging health-care system in Zaire, already crippled by the dramatic impact of AIDS, was confronted with a serious measles epidemic. In 1989, health officials in the capital city of Kinshasa began a vaccination program which, in conjunction with a new system of surveillance and data assessment, had dramatic results. Subsequent examination of data in this city of four million citizens indicated a marked reduction in the number of measles cases among children under age five, while rates of illness from the two other major causes of childhood disease in Zaire—malaria and diarrhea—had not declined.

The use of data in Zaire was facilitated by several factors: There were trained and motivated decisionmakers and technical experts at the national level; data were available from both public health surveillance systems and special studies; priority was given to measles control both locally and internationally; consensus and awareness were developed throughout the health-care delivery system; medical consultation and support were obtained through the international community; there was collaboration among agencies to endorse the concept of the project and facilitate its implementation; and changes were implemented at no increase in cost to the measles-control program in Zaire.

The devastating combination of economic distress and disease in Zaire parallels the crisis facing the City of New York. The basic principles of decision making and policy setting differ very little between Kinshasa and New York City. And New York City has the advantage of tradition and infrastructure to deal with the health crisis confronting its citizens.

What, then, is my vision of implementing data-driven planning for health care in the City of New York? Dr. David Eddy, a well-known health-care analyst, recently developed a health-information planning system he describes as the "War Room for Health." Combining the best available information with the sophistication of computer software and hardware, Eddy conceived a data-driven process that would enable the commissioner of health in a city such as New York to choose rationally among alternatives ranging from clinical delivery of services in hospitals to local immunization programs.

Like the information centers developed by the National Aeronautics and Space Administration for the space shuttle or by the Department of Defense for protection against nuclear attack, various scenarios can be played out based on the best available data and alternative assumptions of effectiveness. Information would be available at the commissioner's desk, the value of which would be limited only by the user friendliness of the software program and the availability of accurate and timely surveillance data combined with data on cost and cost-effectiveness. Such a system would allow the commissioner, the board, and various advisers and consultants to compare the impact of alternative scenarios before making policy. Other relevant issues—such as the preferences of the citizens of New York and judgments on ethics, political realities, and other more qualitative (yet equally important) dimensions of the decision-making process—can be considered in concert with the best available quantitative data.

For example, suppose that in the planning process for 1993, New York City had discretionary funds of $10 million. The commissioner of health, given several alternatives for spending these dollars, could ask: How many lives would be saved through each alternative? How many cases of illness and injury would be prevented? How many dollars would be saved in future years in terms of medical and hospital costs? What would be the long-term return on investment in terms of disability years and its impact on the services of the City of New York?

Is such a system unreasonable? I think not. During "Operation Desert Storm," daily visual communication between troops in the desert and decisionmakers in the Pentagon were conducted through satellite. Using the best available computer systems, various scenarios were played out as new data from the war were provided to the Pentagon. Because health is not given as high a priority as war, the ideal system will not likely be seen in the immediate future. Nevertheless, the tools necessary to establish such a data-driven process are at hand. Eddy has already developed computer models that demonstrate the usefulness of this approach to health policy. He has demonstrated how this system could dramatically change national policy in the area of cholesterol screening for cardiovascular disease, and he is extending his work into other areas of medical care. CDC is currently exploring ways to assess the effectiveness of prevention activities in public health.

While Eddy developed a system for health-care planning, it can easily be used for anticipating the impact of alternative cuts in the budget. Some of the proposed budget cuts for the City of New York would eventually have a devastating impact on health. No sophisticated computer simulations are needed to draw this conclusion. But by using computer simulations, alternative scenarios that minimize the impact on the health of the citizens of New York could be developed under the same budget restrictions to optimize available resources in the health sector. In addition, analysis could forecast the long-term impact of various alternatives and anticipate serious and unacceptable compromises of delivery of curative and preventive services and even collapse of the health-care system in New York City.

New York faces a health emergency comparable to a natural disaster: The reported cases of syphilis, tuberculosis, and acquired immunodeficiency syndrome (AIDS) have been rising at rates higher than those in the entire country. In the past year, there has been a dramatic measles epidemic in the city. There is increasing overcrowding and medical gridlocks in the city's emergency rooms. In the South Bronx, there is a disturbing association between shrinking city services (such as those provided by the fire department) and rising levels of violent deaths, HIV infections, and drug-related illness and death.[1] The differences in the rates of infant and adult mortality between blacks and whites are increasing.[2] (Black men in Harlem are less likely to reach the age of sixty-five than men in Bangladesh.)[3]

In the event of a natural or human-made disaster, epidemiologists often are asked to help assess the health impact, to set up surveillance and emergency triage systems for handling a variety of problems with a minimum of resources. An emergency health team or task force set up at the Department of Health, empowered to acquire data and essential support, would focus available resources on this problem. In a normal situation, we have the luxury of some redundancy and decentralization. In a crisis, no such freedom exists. We must focus our energies on the priority problems of the day. Such an intense look at the City of New York is essential. The Board of Health, the Department of Health, and those who set policy in New York—those who are, ultimately, accountable for the health of all the citizens of New York—need the vision and the will to do this.

I believe that decisions in this arena need to be driven by data, and that the "Data for Decision Making" process will be able to combine societal, political, and ethical parameters with quantitative health data to allow policymakers to set constructive public health goals and to make sound public health decisions.

Several things must be done quickly. First, financial resources must be obtained. New York is facing serious economic constraints; the fiscal resources available to address these public health problems simply are not adequate. Innovative solutions are required. A lesson might be taken from Peru, where, as in Zaire, war and disease have devastated health-care systems and circumstances demand a dramatic response. The devastation brought on by cholera in Peru (and the rest of Latin America) has led the Pan American Health Organization to develop a $50-billion-a-year regional plan for cholera prevention and control. Each country provides 70 percent of the total monies; the remainder is obtained from external sources such as the World Bank. Outside assistance from the private sector also may be a key in New York City.

Second, priorities must be set. This is a very difficult problem, but one that must be faced head on—especially in a city like New York in which resources are increasingly limited. If life expectancy is at the top of the list, then resources might be diverted toward direct patient care (particularly for patients with immediately life-threatening disease). If lower infant mortality is a higher priority, then funds might go instead to prenatal and neonatal care. If keeping adults at work is a top priority, resources might be directed toward occupational health and safety. Or New York City might want to focus its investment on the future, and make its highest priority the prevention of disease and injury of its children.

Of course, New Yorkers want all of these things. But New York is facing a crisis and must compromise. A data-driven decision-making process can, by revealing the consequences of alternative policy decisions on public health, make a significant difference in achieving basic goals.

Oregon has proposed a new approach to priority setting that merits attention. It provides its citizens and professionals with data on effectiveness and cost, and then incorporates public attitudes and values into its process for rationing public funding of health-care dollars.[4] As a result, the state proposes to distribute public funds quite differently from the manner currently mandated by federal law. CDC-sponsored programs in community health planning have demonstrated citizens' ability to grasp and utilize data effectively in looking at policy questions. New York must think creatively and rigorously about how to set priorities in health, including community participation in the decision-making process.

Third, the data that will facilitate the most intelligent decision making on how to achieve whatever priorities are chosen must be identified. Securing the right—and the best available—data is critical to achieving the most effective and efficient public health policy. As priorities crystallize into policies, data collection and analysis will provide timely and accurate indicators of progress in health.

The City of New York faces enormous problems, and solutions are not clear. The citizens of New York must be told that the city's health system is in "imminent peril." Then mechanisms must be developed to deal with the immediate crisis and a system constructed to rebuild and integrate health-care networks at all levels—taking into account the diversity of decisions (including changes in public safety, fire prevention and control, and social services) that have an impact on health.

The concept of a war room for health in New York City is both appropriate and feasible. The basics already exist: the data systems, computer hardware and software, and, most important, the talented men and women. What is needed is leadership, vision, and political will.

A Federal Response

❖ *Congressman Charles Rangel* ❖

A s a politician, I know very well how often we talk about problems and leave our audiences saying, "So, what." They walk away feeling they have not been told anything they did not know before. When is he going to tell us how he is going to solve the problem and what he wants us to do?

We are reaching a stage in our history when politicians better start telling the people what we are going to do to solve the problems for the long run, or our nation just will not be able to face its challenges as we head into the next century. I do not believe that this mandate is any different for public health than it is for the myriad of other problems we face. In fact, I believe that so many of these problems, including public health, are intertwined in such a way that if we do not face them as one problem we will fail or sputter as we have been doing this past decade during the Reagan-Bush years.

Lately, I have been hearing a great deal about the need to be prepared for tomorrow's challenges. The Ways and Means Committee, of which I am a member, has been holding hearings on America's ability to compete in world markets. Generally, I am not terribly excited about hearings focusing on the intricacies of business. But this time I have taken a very considerable interest. I wanted to know what course the Bush administration, our business leaders, and our prominent economists believe the nation must take to be competitive, to maintain our prosperity, and to be able to provide for those less fortunate. The witnesses kept saying that we must invest now to be productive in the future. They were adamant about the failure of having only a short-term view of our problems. They claim that it is American business's, indeed American society's, need for short-term satisfaction in the way of profits or results that has left us with stagnant growth in productivity and problems that appear to be ever-lasting. They claim that without investment today, we will not be able to match our foreign competition tomorrow.

These experts call for the return of capital cost recovery incentives, such as lower capital gains rates and investment tax credits. They seek tax incentives for research and development. In no small way they want the federal government to provide the resources to help them prepare for the future. I sat there at the hearings in a state of chagrin. I have seen the federal government provide all of these incentives, and yet I have not seen the improvements in productivity the business leaders and economists have claimed. What I have not seen is the kind of investment in people that I am confident will have more of a cost-benefit gain than any other if we are to have improving productivity and prosperity.

Constantly, I ask these experts what benefits they see from improving education, health care, and housing for our communities. I ask if they see improvements in productivity if we tap those parts of our communities not now producing, or, in fact, draining our communities' resources. Unfortunately, I usually am the recipient of a muddled answer that indicates our president and his administration and business leaders truly have not recognized the long-term benefits of improving public health, educating all of our young effectively, and providing an opportunity for a decent place to live for *all Americans*.

I have come to the conclusion that we must invest heavily now in the education, health, and shelter of our young Americans if we are to continue to see a prosperous America. I have come to this conclusion after having spent the past several years leading a congressional effort in the war against the most significant public health problem of my congressional district and so many other sections of our city and nation: narcotics. The evidence is clear to me that the scourge of drugs is a public health problem, albeit one of several public health problems our city and nation face. It is a disease that is robbing from our city's and nation's future countless productive citizens and replacing them with enormous burdens on our resources. But it is a problem that is not beyond our ability to resolve.

Narcotics is a case in which the federal government must respond to the nation's public health problems with a long-term view instead of a short-term fix, if it is to promote a high level of national productivity and prosperity. We must strike at the root causes of the narcotics problem, not just its symptoms. While we cannot cease to take legal action against drug dealers and treat those addicted to narcotics, we will never solve the problem until we replace despair with hope. We will not be able to do that unless we recognize the need to provide a healthy environment, education as a vehicle to fulfill expectations, and quality shelter as the haven to nurture the dream. It seems to me that in the long run, the share of our treasury to reach these goals will be cheaper than the millions we spend each year on our police, courts, prisons, and health care for those sicker than they should have been.

There is no question that quality public health is a key element in creating the environment necessary to stem the further deterioration of the community through the cancer of drugs. There is no question in my mind, after twenty-one years in the House of Representatives, that the federal government has a role to play in this effort. In health care, we need a proactive federal government to take leadership not only on insurance for reimbursement but also on the delivery of services, the research of health-care problems, and the environment of poverty.

The strictest definition of public health is the provision of a healthy environment and the control of communicable diseases. I would contend that neither of these goals is achievable unless we solve the biggest public health problems we face today: narcotics, AIDS, and inadequate care for the indigent. Without solving these problems, we in New York City will always be facing a public health problem.

I want to focus here on the role of the federal government and health care. The federal government has been involved in the delivery of health care to the indigent for many years. Medicaid, established in 1975, was supposed to provide sufficient resources to secure quality care for the poor. We all know that that dream has not been realized. Instead, Medicaid has been inadequately funded by both the federal and state governments. Not enough of those who need the program are covered; millions remain uninsured. It has become, in large part, a program to provide a safety net for middle- and working-class families needing expensive long-term care.

Why is this a problem in New York? Over 15 percent of New Yorkers and 33 percent of the city's children depend upon Medicaid, while as many as 20 percent more of the city's population live without any health insurance. In fact, over 40 percent of the Medicaid dollars in New York go to the long-term care of only 11 percent of the beneficiaries. In the meanwhile, the poor are provided with coverage that does not begin to adequately encourage private physicians to provide care, and only allows hospitals to barely eke out their reimbursement.

You may ask, how is this a public health problem? Well, there is clearly a "health deficit" when over 30 percent of those who are poor say their health is poor. There is clearly a public health problem when the emergency rooms of our hospitals are overwhelmed by New Yorkers on Medicaid, uninsured individuals, drug addicts, and AIDS patients. In fact, New Yorkers are using emergency rooms at twice the rate of the rest of America. How does a hospital manage trauma care when its emergency rooms are burdened with primary care cases and cases that have become severe because of the lack of primary care? There is clearly a public health problem when much of our primary health care is provided in the ambulatory units of our hospitals, while state and federal governments—through Medicaid and Medicare—have failed to fully address the millions of dollars of uncompensated care in hospitals and virtually starved hospitals to near bankruptcy. There is clearly a public health problem when the Medicaid system in our city encourages the proliferation of "Medicaid Mills" spreading drug addiction instead of serving the afflicted. It is clearly a problem when the survival rate among males over forty living in Central Harlem is lower than for their counterparts in Bangladesh.

When we look at the poor and their health, the biggest public health-care problem we have is the health of our poor children. If we do not address this problem, we will reap sorrowful burdens later. We already see the results of past neglect in the high level of illness among poor children and their weaker performance in school. Because we neglect poor children and their parents, we are confronted with neonatal intensive care facilities filled with crack and AIDS babies; we are forced to deal with altogether too many brain-injured, lead-poisoned children; we have to deal with infinitely more teenage drug addicts and teenage pregnancies.

I have promised that I would not simply offer you a litany of the problems but would propose what I believe should be the federal response.

The heart of the Reagan-Bush philosophy has been to reduce the role of the federal government and to return to the states and local governments the responsibilities the federal government had been bearing. The only problem is that the states and municipalities have been unable to muster the political support and financial capability to take on these responsibilities. All one has to have seen to understand the difficulties of the states and municipalities are this year's agonizing budget crises of City Hall and Albany as well our neighbors in Connecticut and New Jersey. The Reagan-Bush effort is a cruel and cynical one; it relieves the well-off of their tax burdens and places the burden on the middle and working classes. Instead of using the progressive federal income tax, we now must rely upon the tax structures of the states and

municipalities, whose property and sales taxes are generally regressive and incapable of raising sufficient revenues without undermining the economies of these jurisdictions.

The federal government has played a role in providing insurance for payment for health care through its Medicaid and
Medicare programs; it has, both directly and indirectly (through
mortgage insurance), provided funds for health-care facilities and for traditional public health activities; it has helped
influence the numbers, training, and placement of health-care
professionals; and it has been a major provider of funds for
health research. Unfortunately, the federal government
reduced its role in all of these areas in the 1980s.

If we are to successfully face the challenges of the next century, the federal government must increase spending in all
these areas. We need not create new programs. Current programs, which work well when funded, and reform of the health
insurance system should make the difference. Further, these
are cost-effective expenditures; they will reduce expenditures
in many areas in future years.

To a large extent over the past decade, federal funding for
public health-related programs has declined (when adjust-
ed for inflation). Several programs have seen real cuts. While
others have seen increases, funding has not grown as fast as
the need. For example, federal funding of community health
centers—one of the few sources of health care in communities such as mine—has only increased by a third over a
decade in which inflation surely outstripped need.

The National Health Service Corps, designed to provide
scholarships for the medical education of those dedicated to
serving the poor, has been cut by two-thirds since 1980.
There were 1,600 participants in the program in 1985, but only
135 in 1990, while there were requests for over 1,000 vacan-
cies. The program once had enough participants to provide
additional professionals for such institutions as Harlem
Hospital. Now there are so few participants that African-
American physicians participating in the programs who

hoped to practice in the inner city have been posted to where the need is even more dire: Indian reservations.

Another area subject to severe cuts has been support for public health administration. The federal effort in this area has been cut (in absolute dollars) by over 50 percent. Similarly, the Preventive Health Block Grant program has seen a cut (in absolute dollars) of over 50 percent.

There have been exceptions. Considerable increases in spending, which reflect growing needs, have occurred in programs fighting AIDS, in programs combating drug and alcohol abuse, and in programs providing immunizations.

There is no question that the combination of Medicaid and Medicare has made a significant contribution to public health. Unfortunately, even as the outlays for both programs have spiraled beyond the imagination of their creators, they have not kept pace with the costs of health care. Every year, for the past several years, the administration has tried to cut the growth of these programs to where providers are pinched and beneficiaries are experiencing real pain. Congress has usually restored a substantial amount of the cuts and has tried to balance program growth with reasonable cost control. The impact has lessened the ability of hospitals to function effectively and physicians to continue serving covered patients.

This year, our hospitals are confronted with new regulations that affect the reimbursement of their capital expenditures under the Medicare system. The purpose of the new reimbursement scheme is to discourage unnecessary capital expenditures and to improve the occupancy rates of hospitals. New York hospitals already operate at about the highest occupancy rates of any in the nation. Further, New York hospitals have either recently undergone modernization programs or will very shortly undertake them, totaling well into billions of dollars. The reimbursement scheme proposed by the federal authorities seriously jeopardizes our hospitals and their ability to service their debt and operate their facilities. This is frightening when we are relying on hospitals to provide basic care to so many underserved communities.

New regulations changing the method for reimbursing physicians will have the effect of reducing the Medicare reimbursement for Manhattan-based physicians by as much as 30 percent. This cutback could make it difficult for many physicians and clinics to continue to serve elderly patients and to take on new Medicare patients.

Why have we abandoned our effort to make these programs work?

Have we decided that there is no need for more community health centers? In the north end of my congressional district, there is Presbyterian Hospital. It has admirably tried to provide the community with ambulatory care in the face of huge losses over the past several years. But Presbyterian cannot alone meet the needs of the community, and they have asked me to help them secure federal funds for a community health center much like the William F. Ryan Center on the West Side. I had to tell them that there might just be enough money for one center per state, and they would have to compete with worthy applications throughout the state. But we should be looking to provide community health centers wherever there is a shortage of primary care. More centers would mean lower Medicaid costs, lower emergency room costs, and a healthier, more productive community. We should restore funding for community health centers to the early 1980s level.

Likewise, I cannot understand why it has taken so long for Congress to recognize its mistake in cutting the National Health Service Corps. Congress has recently authorized a restoration of the program. Congress should appropriate enough funds to provide enough physicians not only for Indian reservations but also for rural areas and inner cities.

We must increase our spending on both drug addiction prevention and treatment. There have been increases, but this is clearly one of the greatest public health problems we face. I am convinced that money spent on these programs will result in great savings for the criminal justice system and the health-care system. Does it pay to spend money now on an at-risk teenager or an addict or to spend $30,000 per year later to keep that person in prison?

Health research is important as well. True, we have increased research into AIDS. But we need to do more research in many areas. We need to continue work in traditional areas and to increase funds for research into new areas, such as how life-style affects health.

We have to face the fact that relying on current private health insurance and the Medicaid scheme simply is not working. We all know the number of uninsured Americans: thirty-seven million and growing. In New York City, 20 percent of the population is without health insurance. For children, the statistics are even worse: 23 percent are uninsured. There is no question in my mind that this results in inadequate care and reduced public health. It results in people not being able to afford regular health care and suffering for it. It results in many communities lacking physicians. We would not have to worry about inadequate Medicaid payments and uncompensated care if we had a national health insurance plan. It would mean that hospitals could appropriately budget. It would mean that it could be economically possible to practice medicine in places like Central Harlem. It would mean that people would see physicians before they became too sick.

There are several plans being proposed—from an extension of Medicare to the Canadian All-Payer plan to a play-or-pay plan. Congressman Dan Rostenkowksi, chairman of the House Ways and Means Committee, has just proposed a play-or-pay proposal that would require businesses to provide a minimum health insurance plan for employees or pay into a pool to support insurance for the remaining population. Under this plan, Medicaid would be expanded, and Medicare eligibility would begin at age sixty. I have cosponsored a plan introduced by Congressman Marty Russo of Chicago. It is patterned after the Canadian plan. I prefer to replace the current scheme, especially Medicaid, with one basic plan that covers everyone equally, funded with progressive taxes. I believe that such a plan would supply the framework for the type of cooperation between government and health-care providers that can keep costs in check and still meet the reasonable needs of those providing the services, the pharmaceuticals, and the other medical supplies.

It is clear that the road to a national health insurance plan must pass through three stages. First, there must be a national consensus that there is a need for reform. Such a consensus now exists. Nearly every segment of the society and the economy that has a stake in health care recognizes the need for reform. Second, there must be a political consensus as to what course should be taken. I believe we are in the midst of this stage. But we will remain in this stage until the one official who is elected by all the people comes forth with his proposal. Until President Bush has the courage to face the American people with a proposal that will become the focus of debate there can be no progress to the remaining stage and resolution to an effective program.

Unfortunately, we have a president who has no vision for domestic policy and the needs of the American people. He has little or no comprehension of the health needs of the great mass of America. And he certainly has no idea of the depth of the health problems of the inner city. Finally, should the president show some leadership, a consensus will be necessary on how to pay for the agreed-upon plan. If the nation can navigate this road, we may well have a plan in place later on in this decade. I am certain it will change the nature of the public health picture as it will change for the better the health-care system of the nation.

I may be too optimistic about where we can go. Maybe I should not be optimistic. So much of what must be done is not being done by the federal government because we have painted ourselves into a corner with the budget and legislation that has taken away our prerogatives. But my constituents have given me the mandate and freedom to speak out and to defy the current budget conventions. When it comes to public health and all that it means I will speak out. I will do all I can to prod the federal government to move forward to insuring the health of all Americans, regardless of their wealth or whether they have health insurance. We can afford to do no less if we are going to insure our future.

Crisis and Cooperation

❖ *Mayor David N. Dinkins* ❖

Today, New York City faces a health-care crisis of staggering proportions. The magnitude of the problem is severe: At a time when the federal government has abandoned our cities and New York is battling a national and regional recession, our most vulnerable residents simply do not have access to the high-quality primary and preventive health care they need. Instead, many New Yorkers are forced to rely on hospital emergency rooms as their sole source of health care. And some 1.3 million men, women, and children in New York City are without health insurance. Many have never seen a doctor in their entire lives.

As a result, we face tremendous challenges in our public health system. The statistics are horrifying. Infant mortality in New York City is one-third higher than the national average—and the rate for African Americans is *twice* as high as that for whites. A large percentage of pregnant women in New York City receive prenatal care only late in pregnancy—if at all. Maternal drug use has risen by more than 300 percent in the past few years.

I will share with you some other statistics, because these numbers paint the barren landscape that public health officials are now facing. Clearly, the most devastating public health crisis of the 1990s is the epidemic of HIV, the virus that causes AIDS. Over 34,000 AIDS cases have been reported in New York City, and our Department of Health projects that we can expect 36,000 new cases between 1991 and 1995. And that's only the tip of the iceberg. Between 125,000 and 235,000 individuals in the city are believed to be HIV-infected but not yet experiencing full-blown AIDS.

Many diseases once thought to be eradicated are again at epidemic levels. Tuberculosis, an ancient scourge that was proclaimed near death a few years ago, has taken on a fierce new life. Cases of tuberculosis rose 132 percent between 1980 and 1990—38 percent from 1989 to 1990 alone. This accounts for 15 percent of the nation's reported cases in that period. Last year, there were 2,400 reported measles cases in New York City. In the first six months of this year, there have already been 3,500 reported cases. And the consequences have been especially severe for people of color—and for recent immigrants, many of whom are not aware of the importance and availability of immunizations.

And sadly, in this time of extraordinary need, primary care doctors and nurses and other allied health workers are in short supply. The past few months have been very difficult for every one of us. A crippling fiscal crisis has forced us to cut back and even eliminate valued programs. In these extraordinarily demanding fiscal times, we have had to look at what is most essential and make some very difficult policy decisions. I had to make some of the hardest choices of my mayoralty, choices that caused me tremendous personal pain, as I was forced—because of the $3.5 billion budget gap we had to close—to cut programs that I know protect the public health of this city.

But through some very hard work in those agonizing final days of the budget process, we were able to find the revenue to restore a great deal of money to the health programs we could least afford to lose. I am particularly proud of the restorations we have made to programs that affect the future of our city—our children. We were able to restore funding to critical programs such as our infant mortality initiative, the bureau of day care inspections, the bureau of immunizations, and school health services. We were also able to restore much-needed dollars to our tuberculosis program.

Of course, despite these restorations, we are continuing our crusade to make our health-care programs more efficient and more effective as we enter the twenty-first century—and continuing our efforts to downsize government without compromising the quality of services—in health care and in all areas. Toward that end, I have appointed a special task force of city commissioners, led by First Deputy Mayor Norman Steisel, and complemented by our Management Advisory Task Force of government, business, and labor leaders, which is taking a close look at the city's overall system of health-service delivery. Within that context, we are paying special attention to the City's Health Department, which is truly at the forefront of national public health policy, to determine what its primary goals and focus must be in the coming century. In a few months, I will receive the task force's recommendations on ways we can further downsize, consolidate, and improve our health services and policy.

But city government alone cannot fight these problems. We need to join forces in a coalition—a coalition of community organizations, service providers, the private sector, and the state and federal governments—if we are to truly meet our health challenges. We must begin to exchange ideas, mobilize our resources, and work *together* to implement a health-care strategy for the coming decades.

We are working to attract the attention of the federal government to issues of health care. If the federal government had maintained the level of aid it gave New York City ten years ago, our operating budget would have received an additional $1.2 billion this year, and a substantial proportion of that would have been directed to health and human services.

But it is not just New York City that feels the pain of the federal government's abandonment—this crisis is not unique to one city, or even to urban areas. It extends throughout the United States. This country spends a higher percentage of its gross national product on health care than any other industrialized nation, yet many of our people are still unable to receive the care they so desperately need.

The growth of our uninsured population is of particular concern: thirty-seven million Americans have no health insurance. One out of five New Yorkers under age eighteen is without any health coverage—neither Medicaid nor private insurance. For New York State alone, that means that 700,000 children who lack coverage face a major impediment in receiving appropriate medical services. As a result, many hospitals have essentially become the family doctor for the poor. This is an issue that demands solutions on a national level—the federal government simply *must* address this inadequate coverage—along with the inadequacy of Medicaid and Medicare treatment.

This appalling lack of preventive and primary care in communities throughout the nation—a shortage for which our hospitals, without adequate resources, are left to compensate—also demands the attention of every level of government. But in the meantime, we can begin on the local level. Here in New York, one solution lies in harnessing the coordinated efforts of our city's business, medical, and government sectors and forming partnerships that will work within our communities to address their needs. The themes of partnership and of community-based services have been the guiding principles of my administration, and our approach promises much success in the arena of health.

We must signal a new era of collaboration and provide forums for the development of creative solutions to address the most critical health issues of our day. Only by working together as partners can we combat a health crisis that is draining the energy of our people and tearing at the very fabric that holds our communities together. But our entire country feels the pain of inadequate health care, and I am calling on President Bush to join our coalition in a meaningful way, with resources and technology. He can begin by supporting a system of national health care that ensures equal access to quality care for all Americans.

For while the federal contribution has been shrinking, the problems we face in public health have been growing by leaps and bounds. A decade ago, only a handful of cases of AIDS had been reported. Crack had not yet hit the streets. Tuberculosis, syphilis, and measles were viewed as diseases of a bygone era.

The sad irony is that these *could* have been problems of a bygone era if Washington had given them the same kind of attention and priority as, for example, the Savings and Loan bailout or the war in the Persian Gulf. And despite the fact that we have just experienced the worst epidemic of measles in almost two decades—a disease that is completely preventable through appropriate immunization—the president did not push to adopt a plan to provide emergency funds for the vaccinations that would swiftly curb outbreaks of this disease. Rather, this kinder, gentler president chose to send a team of senior officials and health experts to six cities across the nation "to learn why kids aren't getting immunized."

We don't need a special task force to answer that question. The answer is simple—the lack of an adequate health-care system and the gutting of the federal program for child immunization over the past decade. The Bush administration has launched a campaign to eradicate tuberculosis by the year 2010, and yet has allocated a paltry $12 million for tuberculosis-control programs throughout the entire nation. Sad to say that we could use all that money for tuberculosis control right now, right here in New York City.

As for the State of New York, like us, the state is in a serious fiscal crisis, and, like us, the state has had to make some serious cuts to health-care services. But Governor Cuomo and I have made a commitment to work more closely together, to combine our limited resources, and to look for more creative ways to approach our serious health problems.

For example, I recently signed a New York/New York agreement with Governor Cuomo to launch an innovative measles-prevention campaign. Under this agreement, city and state agencies will provide immunizations, education, and outreach where they are needed most—in the communities. It will link children with ongoing primary health care, to address the full range of health problems that affect them.

The community also has a role—and a stake—in solving our health-care problems. Any meaningful change requires that government tap the energy and ideas of groups and individuals who work at the community level and are closest to the problems. Community residents and community-based organizations must be directly and actively involved. We need them to help us ensure that the programs and services we provide are sensitive to community needs and concerns.

At the same time, we are working very aggressively to contain our city's growing health-care costs while *improving* the quality of care that we can offer in our communities. One way to do that is through a program of "managed Medicaid"— by linking our most vulnerable residents to a single health-care provider who can offer comprehensive and ongoing health care. This way, we can ensure that people do not have to rely on emergency rooms as their only source of primary care.

Currently, about 38,000 New Yorkers—or 3 percent of the city's Medicaid recipients—are voluntarily enrolled in managed-care programs. And we are starting a pilot program of managed Medicaid in southwest Brooklyn, which will add an additional 30,000 people to this critical initiative. As many of you know, the state has just passed a Managed Medicaid bill, and we are working very hard to develop a citywide plan to reach the enrollment targets that have been established by this important legislation.

I cannot emphasize enough that we are interested in managed Medicaid not solely for its cost saving—although that is certainly important. We are implementing this program mainly because we want to ensure better access to primary health care where it is needed most—in the community. And as we contain our growing Medicaid costs, we also intend to work with the state to find a realistic way to shift the burden of those costs to Albany, so that New York State— like forty-five other states in this country—can do its fair share.

So although our fiscal situation has forced us to make some painful but unavoidable reductions in services, we in government are striving to accomplish more with the resources we have. And when brighter days emerge—and they *will* emerge—I believe that our government will be stronger, more creative, more productive, and more responsive than ever before.

Public Health:
Old Truths, New Realities

❖ *Governor Mario M. Cuomo* ❖

Political leaders are currently faced with having to make budgets under extraordinarily difficult circumstances, with the need and demand for public services growing and our public resources dwindling—eaten away, as we all know, by a national recession and other phenomena. Most of the public all the while is demanding more, and much of the public is needing more, while we are having to say "No" more than we want to.

I think that mayors and governors across the country can appreciate a story, an old story, that they tell about Abraham Lincoln. During the Civil War, when Lincoln was being badgered by all his generals and staff for more support, more men, more money, and he had to say "No" over and over, he contracted, suddenly, a mild case of smallpox. His doctors insisted that he stay quarantined, in bed. Lincoln insisted on going to his office. In explaining his eagerness to go to the office, Lincoln said the following, "At last, I have something I can give everybody." That was Abraham Lincoln.

Since Lincoln's time, it's appropriate to note, we have eliminated smallpox and, for all practical purposes in this country, a number of other public health threats like cholera and typhoid fever and dysentery. It's also appropriate to note that it was here in this city, barely a century ago, that the American public health movement was born to the great and lasting benefit of New Yorkers and of all Americans. But today there are new threats and some recrudescences of old ones attacking the health of the people.

To speak about public health is to speak in truisms, which the dictionary says are "self-evident truths too obvious for mention." There's a danger latent in that kind of obviousness. The current crises and epidemics that are the proximate cause of this book are a warning to us about truisms. A warning about what happens when we are seduced into neglecting truths because of what we take to be their obviousness. A warning that, like our liberty, the truisms that have been the basis of public health policy for almost a century require our constant vigilance. They cannot be taken for granted without risking peril.

I would like to focus briefly on two truisms—old truths, obvious truths that we need to reapply to the new realities that challenge us today. And then about how we have succeeded in applying them, where we have failed, what we need to do in order to fulfill government's obligation to help improve the condition of people's lives.

Truism #1: *An ounce of prevention is worth a pound of cure.* That, it seems to me, is *the* fundamental tenet of the public health credo. So obvious that no one disputes it. Unfortunately, however, we've too frequently honored this precept more with lip service than with action. Measles, syphilis, tuberculosis— all have one thing in common. They are preventable. With proper and available public health measures in place, none should exist in our state today. Yet despite our antibiotic arsenal, we have a resurgence of venereal disease and tuberculosis. Measles, which we thought we were on the verge of eliminating, is now stalking the children of our inner city.

AIDS is similar in many respects. Despite some real progress in our understanding of this immensely complex syndrome, there is no known cure for AIDS once it takes hold. We're hopeful, of course, there will be. That's why New York was the first to allocate funds for AIDS research. Since 1983, we've committed more than $19 million to that effort—just part of our overall commitment of more than $1 billion of state funds to combat AIDS. But while scientists struggle to find a cure for AIDS, there are things that we could be doing to prevent its spread. Right now.

Remember the story of John Snow, who, in 1853, left an enduring lesson in epidemiology and public health. He found that all the victims of a cholera epidemic then sweeping through parts of London, drank water from one particular pump on Broad Street. He removed the handle of the Broad Street pump and put an end to the epidemic thirty years before the causative agent of cholera was isolated by Robert Koch.

We're trying to do something analogous with AIDS. We know some of the ways it is transmitted—through certain sexual practices and other habits such as the sharing of needles among intravenous drug users. In New York, we have a massive educational campaign to inform people, especially those in the high-risk groups, about the danger of engaging in those practices. We're trying to do what John Snow did—stop it even if we can't yet cure it.

Preventive strategies didn't work—because they were not applied or were ignored—for 1,200 babies born with congenital syphilis last year, or for the 3,500 children who contracted measles this year, or for the more than 4,000 people infected with tuberculosis, or for the 35,000 children and adults in our state we know have AIDS.

The result of all of this is needless suffering, even death. A terrible loss of potential and, beyond that, a terrible cost to all of us in expensive treatment and hospitalization that could have been avoided, and that's the part that hurts.

The state has joined with the city in a "New York/New York" agreement to halt the measles epidemic. Instead of acting like separate entities trying to solve many of the same problems separately, state and city agencies, with the assistance of community organizations, will pool their efforts through this agreement to immunize 50,000 preschool children in those neighborhoods with a high incidence of measles.

Major initiatives are also under way to deal with the other current epidemics. For tuberculosis, diagnostic services are being extended to reach the homeless, and treatment is being carefully monitored to assure that each patient completes the full course of antibiotic therapy. To combat syphilis, testing is being conducted in all hospitals, family planning clinics, drug treatment units, and jails in the epidemic communities.

To deal with the AIDS epidemic, we've adopted a five-year plan, a key component of which is the development of "community need profiles," which are used in designing prevention activities for particular communities.

Prevention is, of course, the preferred strategy in any number of areas:

- ☐ In an effort to prevent serious injuries and fatalities, we were the first state in the union to mandate the use of seat belts. The first. The others very swiftly followed.

- ☐ To combat the public health hazards caused by smoking, we passed one of the nation's most effective and far-reaching antismoking statutes to protect nonsmokers. This forceful action is one of many tributes to one of the great health commissioners of all time in this nation's history, Dr. David Axelrod.

- ☐ To help prevent chronic illnesses and disabilities—including cerebral palsy, retardation, autism, and learning disabilities—we've expanded access to prenatal care, especially for those women who previously fell between the cracks, who were not poor enough to qualify for Medicaid but were not able to afford private insurance.

Prevention works. It's an old truth we're trying in a number of ways to reapply to our public health strategies.

But we need to go beyond reaffirming that simple truth. We need to rebuild our public health infrastructure, which brings us to *Truism #2: No man is an island.* No man, no woman, no child is an island, either.

It's also a truth that has been recognized in public health for a long time—that illness does not occur in a vacuum, that the roots of illness are usually deeply implanted in homelessness, in poverty, in other persistent social ills.

The current epidemics are concentrated in communities that are marked by poverty, inadequate health services, jobless-ness, overcrowding, substandard housing, and—most impor-tant—widespread use of illicit drugs.

Health, perhaps more than any other aspect of our lives, depends upon the interconnectedness of everything else we are and do. The very word "health" has the same root as "whole." It denotes an integrity based upon the immense-ly complex synergy that includes the workings of the human body and all the external forces that affect it. Health is not given, nor taken away, in a vacuum.

Our approach to reform in public health, then, must be syn-ergistic to be intelligent. It should mean applying *all* of our strengths to all of our vulnerabilities simultaneously. And it's clear, in public health, that our strengths are not *just* physi-cians, not *just* hospitals, not *just* the amazing array of high-technology, diagnostic tools and curative procedures avail-able to us today.

History teaches us that it is not through medicine *alone* that we can promote better health. As Dr. Lewis Thomas point-ed out, many of the major achievements of the past centu-ry—for example, the elimination in our country of typhoid fever, cholera, and dysentery as deadly diseases—did not hap-pen "because of medicine, or medical science, or the presence of doctors." "Much of the credit should go," Dr. Thomas has said, "to the plumbers and engineers of the Western world."

Today, as then, there is a need in public health policy for a synergistic approach. For medical services, of course. And for a whole range of other services that are tailored to spe-cific community needs, identified by members of the com-munity. That's what our state program, called here in New York "Neighborhood-based Initiative," seeks to accomplish. Synergism.

There's a need for primary care that involves community citizens as health workers, and that takes full advantage of a whole range of professionals working as a team—doctors, nurses, nurse practitioners, physician assistants, health educators, home-care technicians, and others. Primary care that is not episodic and hit-or-miss; that makes the patients—not the professionals—the center of attention; that is coordinated and accessible and accountable. In brief, the kind of care that most of us are able to demand for ourselves and our children. That's what our managed-care initiative is about.

But as important as medicine and medical care are to health status, they are not enough. There's an equal need for a realignment of our priorities so that the opportunities we Americans speak grandly of are *in fact* open to all; so that more people have access to them and a chance to lift themselves out of poverty—a chance to work; to educate themselves; to live in safe, decent housing; to provide themselves and their children adequate, nutritious food.

We all know that the relationship between illness, sickness, and physical frailty on the one hand, and poverty on the other, is not just a grotesque coincidence. It is causal. It is real. It is historic.

We all know that we might have predicted the escalation of ill health from the parallel statistics showing the growth of poverty in this nation and the widening gaps between the minority population at the bottom of the economic ladder and the rest of America. There is a relationship. Cancer, cardiovascular disease, chemical dependency, diabetes, infant mortality—even homicide—we know they are all manifestations of one pathology. We know that they are all, in one way or another, expressions of the ravages and deprivations, the despair and the rage, that are parts of the plight of being poor in America in the last decades of this century.

In New York, the synergistic approach to public health has included our Decade of the Child agenda, and much more. We've had the largest affordable housing program in the country. That relates to health. Acid rain legislation that could serve as a model for the country. That certainly does as well. Exemplary laws to protect men and women in the workplace. A state supplemental nutrition program. A state program to help elderly people get the medications they need but couldn't afford. We've done a lot. Realizing the need for a synergistic approach.

Is it enough? We're shamefully short of where we should be for all we have done. I don't think there's a state in the Union that's much ahead of us in any of these areas. But we are all shamefully behind. That's clear to us and to all of you. Especially clear here in New York City, because everything—both good and bad—tends to be magnified in this great place.

But consider this: Most of the challenges we face, the challenges for this city or our state, are national challenges as well, aren't they? There are more than thirty million Americans with no health insurance, and tens of millions more who are maybe a pink slip away from losing their insurance. There are twenty-three million illiterates who can't read the label on a bottle of poison. We have a national addiction to drugs. This is the issue I wish the American people would focus on because it teaches us so much about the relationship between the national and local governments and the failure of the national part of the partnership.

The difference between my generation and this one? Harry Belafonte and I were in Harlem about a year ago to talk to a group of Decade of the Child children—children we were acknowledging in a special way because they had overcome the impediments and the difficulties of their surroundings and were on their way to great, full, and even inspiring lives in some cases. And Harry got up and said, "You know, I'm right from this area. This is where I came from and we know the problems you have. Mario is from South Jamaica, and boy, that is a tough neighborhood. He had problems just like me and just like you. So we're all in this together."

And I got up and said, "I love Harry and he is one of the brightest people I know. But I have to disagree with him. My time was nothing like your time. We didn't have anything like the problems you have. We had marijuana. We had bad stuff. I'll concede that. But we didn't have coke and we didn't have crack and we didn't have heroin."

And now you have heroin and coke and crack and ice and all these things, most of which you cannot produce in Queens or Harlem. They all come from somewhere else. They are quintessentially international and national. If ever there was a syndrome that plagues us that is not local, it is drugs. It comes past your army, your navy, your secret service, your marines, your diplomats, your $1.5 trillion budget. Nothing stops it, and when it makes it to Queens or the Bronx or Manhattan, you're finished. You can't prevent it with your police. It's here and you're gone and the whole chain starts—the police and the courts and the jails and the probation and the parole and the treatment.

And the federal government announces that it has declared war on drugs, and does it with all the passion and strength of a declaration of war on Saddam Hussein or Adolf Hitler. It says, "This is threat number one to this nation." Announcing thereby that it is indeed quintessentially a national issue. Why else would you declare war from Washington? And then having declared war, they announced: "We neglected to point out to you we cannot afford any troops. This is a different kind of national concern."

We notice children of children in the street. It is killing them as surely as if you took a Scud missile and dropped it on PS 167. It is maybe even worse than a Scud missile, because then at least they would go all at once. But to take even a little at a time, and taking chunks out of them, you're making all of us watch it happen to them. You're making them see it happen to themselves.

We'll raise taxes to meet these needs and others like them, raise them to the point that everyone will mock us and call us neosocialists. We'll be so reckless in the attempt that the experts who mark you for your fiscal prudence will put us on the edge of disappearing ratings. What alternative do we have when this national concern is neglected by the national forces?

But when we plead to the federal government for a little help—not everything, we're willing to do our share—it only makes it worse to be told over and over, "We know you're right but we can't afford to take care of it." It only makes it worse when you are told that in 1983, 1984, and 1985, and the graphs are going up and the deaths are going up and the prison cells are going up at $130,000 apiece, $30,000 to maintain them. When you're going broke in 1987 and 1988 and 1989 and all of a sudden they invest in Savings and Loans . . . after being told year after year that there is no money.

You're in the White House with all the other governors, and they say: "You have to understand, governor. We know you make a very good case. Indeed, you make it eloquently. We can tell you're serious."

"Well, thanks a lot."

"But we just don't have the wealth."

And then all of a sudden you find $50 billion and then $60 billion and $70 billion. And you ask the geniuses who can count, "How did you do that, just so I can explain it to my people; because I made the mistake of going back and saying we don't have the wealth. We have the will, but not the wallet—that's what I said—please tell me what to say to them now. What do I say to them? That I heard you wrong? That you hit a horse? Where did you get this money?"

"This is different. This is off budget."

"That's terrific. That's exactly what I would explain to the people of the state. That this is off budget."

Now if you did that in your drugstore, you would go to jail when the IRS caught you. Off budget means you put it in another category where you wouldn't have to explain it.

You see, in the end, it's all a matter of priorities. You have a hurricane and an earthquake—I know about them both. We were the first in Puerto Rico with our Air National Guard. And the governor, Rafael Hernandez Colon, came here to give us thanks for having recognized what happened there. And the terrible earthquake in California we all saw on television.

It was awful. And when they said they needed $5 billion, they went to the floor of the House and they went to the floor of the Senate and they got $5 billion. I'm not begrudging the $5 billion, but do you know what we could do for a billion dollars in this state? And for $2 billion in the whole nation?

What shall I tell my people? What shall I tell the children? How do I get it straight? How do I get it straight for myself so that I don't just get angry? Or mad with confusion. What do I say then?

Well, it's clear. It's always been clear. It's clear in your own home . . . it's clear in your own office . . . in your own classroom . . . in your own checkbook. You look at the amount of wealth you have available to you and you spend it on the things that are most important. And you choose Savings and Loans and the hurricane and the earthquake and all the other things in this budget . . . an arsenal to fight wars that may have become passé. You chose all of that before addicted children and there is no way around it. That is what you decided.

Now why you decided it, only God and maybe a very clever political consultant can tell you. But that is the truth of it. This is a national issue. It is a national epidemic. Homelessness is a national problem. Nobody does for the homeless what we do. We don't give enough. The federal government does not give enough.

Thirteen million American children trapped in poverty are a national concern. Not a Tennessee concern . . . not an Idaho concern . . . or a New York State concern. A national concern. But over the past decade we've not acted as a nation in dealing with these challenges. Instead, Washington shifted the responsibility toward the states and cities at the same time it withdrew the help it used to give the states and cities.

Mayor Dinkins and I earlier today were at a home for the homeless who happened to have mental illnesses. I wish that all of you had been there with us. It was wonderful to be in these residences, to be with these people, watching them embrace the mayor and kiss the mayor—having them all come up to you and say, "This is wonderful being here. Now we have a bed." Having a woman about sixty-five years old come up and say, "I have a bathroom, let me show you." They made David and me take pictures next to the toilet because they were so delighted at having a bathroom, having a toilet. And David got up and said, "This is wonderful . . . this is a partnership of the state and the city . . . see how we work together."

But then we had to remind ourselves that not everyone does, that there is one partner missing. David and I are very close. You know why? Because we're out there in the cold, freezing. Washington kicked us out and said, "You guys are on your own." That's why we're so close together—we were kicked out of the same house. We're dealing with the same wants . . . feeling the same loneliness. Housing was cut about 80 percent. Energy conservation, 67 percent. Job training, 65 percent. Revenue sharing gone. Urban development grants gone. Money for education, environment, mass transit all cut.

Synergism. This is all relevant to public health. These cuts have had an immense impact. You know what it means today to David Dinkins's budget. In New York City, the decade-long federal withdrawal has added $2 billion to this city's budget gap. In other words, even if you hadn't made a whole lot of progress, but just stayed where we were, David wouldn't have all this heat, all this aggravation . . . all this confusion . . . all this pain. He'd have the $2 billion he needs for his budget. That's what this federal withdrawal means.

I'm complaining, yes. I'm saying it every chance I get, and so is David, and we're going to say it more and more and more and more. When people talk about "the failure of the cities" and about "failed liberal policies," we'll explain whose failure it is, where drugs really come from, and who has a responsibility for education.

I'll talk to you about failure. Think about this: The best thing you've been able to do for four years is win a war; the best thing you've been able to boast of is destroying 100,000 lives and dropping bombs down smokestacks. Think of this: You want to talk about failure, you can't stand up and say to the American people, "I gave you better health. I gave you more housing; I helped you build roads and bridges; I helped you to educate yourself; I lifted your children from the ghettos and gave you the same kind of opportunity I had." You cannot say that.

What you can say is "I won the war." Well, you might have won one war. You didn't win the war in the streets. That's what New York City is, and New York City is not just New York City. New York City is America, because there are people like this all over the United States of America. The difference between us and most of the rest of the country is that we live in tighter quarters. You pack twelve million people a day in one place in New York City, you see everything magnified. But this is America. All of it . . . the rich, the poor, the illiterate. We see it all at once in New York City.

We need a whole lot of things. You know what they are. We need a national Decade of the Child. We need to fund the Women, Infants and Children Program and fully fund Head Start. Do you know what Head Start is? Do you want to talk about health? Want to talk about putting kids into a position where they could learn what they should do for themselves? Look at any of the charts of kids who had Head Start and kids who didn't have Head Start. They make so much more headway.

How could you not invest fully in that program when you did a $1.5 trillion of other things? When you took the wealthiest people in the world—some of them—and took their taxes from 70 percent for unearned and 50 percent for earned and reduced it all the way to 28. Incidentally, when you started talking about cutting, you said we'll settle for 40, but you like the idea of freeing up the wealth so much you went all the way down to 28. Until now you are the least heavily taxed industrial nation in the world, and Japan writes books about you. They say, "What a bunch of crybabies you are. You blow the money back to the rich people and then you complain about us doing better than you. You don't want to invest in yourself." With all of that I'm unhappy when you tell us that you don't have enough money to put into the Head Start program. It doesn't make any sense.

Finally, we have to enlarge our national vision to include everybody, all that you need to include, to get the kind of synergism that's necessary. Include the lucky and the left-out, include the young and the old, inner-city kids and wealthy suburbanites; the well-read and the illiterate; the millions seeking drug treatment; the millions more seeking only a chance to grow and learn and make their own way. Why don't we recognize that they're all a part of one world and deal with all of them? We need to enlarge our national vision—not just as an act of compassion, but because our national economic self-interest demands that we do.

A physician-poet put all of this in words more eloquent than any I have. His name is familiar to you, I'm sure: William Carlos Williams. He was a family doctor who practiced in a small New Jersey community for more than forty years, and he also happened to be one of America's most powerful poetic voices. As a doctor, he faced the palpable mysteries of life and death, as many of you do as daily parts of your working lives. And as a poet, he searched out the limits and the essences of the American character, trying to understand through his writing what makes us what we are as a people.

Once he was asked why he hadn't gone off to Europe like so many of the other American artists and writers of his time. He said straight out, "Because the world force is here in America. We have something all our own. Something vital and alive and new. And we must work with it, use it, celebrate it." His questioner seemed puzzled, asked him to explain this world force. He said, "We're still creating the future by dreaming it first, and it's something we're dreaming together." That was the world force William Carlos Williams struggled to see beneath the hard, often unloving facts of everyday life—a dream, "a dream that doesn't leave anyone out."

Like many of you, I know how powerfully this city has nurtured dreams. I have told stories over and over of being born ten miles from here and growing up above a grocery store, and how a generation later my mother, my family, attended my eldest daughter's graduation from medical school. I remember my mother crying and saying, a bit prematurely, "My God, my granddaughter is a doctor." Talk about dreams fulfilled.

Like many of you, when I look back on my life in this city all I can say is, "My God, how good this city has been to me, to us, to my family and to so many of my friends." But I think that recognition is an inadequate response to our good luck unless it leads us to work so that new seekers of dreams can have their day as well. The state will extend itself to see that that happens.

Conclusion

❖ *Kevin M. Cahill, M.D.* ❖

New York has been the cradle for many, if not most, of the public health programs and policies that are now accepted as part of the American way of life. It is not surprising, therefore, that there are important lessons the whole nation must learn from the near disaster that recently challenged the oldest and most preeminent department of health in the nation.

The delivery of health services in the next decade will dominate the domestic political arguments in America. It is painfully obvious that public health is one of the indispensable foundations of our entire social system. One cannot rationally tackle the complex issues of poverty, housing, education, or welfare, much less the specific problems of addiction, health insurance, or access to care while silently watching the public health system crumble because of a distorted set of government priorities, mismanagement, or a tragic case of gross neglect.

This volume offers historical, legal, economic, political, and moral bases for reconstructing an essential part of the American dream. Our leaders must understand the necessity for public health programs, and appreciate their importance in maintaining a safe and civilized society. An enlightened and aroused citizenry must be vigilant in demanding that the *imminent peril* that faced New York City in the summer of 1991 never again be allowed to slip silently into a destructive reality.

About the Authors

Kevin M. Cahill, M.D. is the Senior Member of the New York City Board of Health. He is also Clinical Professor of Public Health at the University of New Jersey College of Medicine, Director of the Tropical Disease Center at Lenox Hill Hospital in New York, and Professor and Chairman of International Health at the Royal College of Surgeons in Ireland. He has also served as Chairman of the New York State Health Planning Commission, the New York State Health Research Council, and as Assistant to the Governor of New York for Health Affairs.

The Honorable Mario M. Cuomo is serving his third term as the Chief Executive of New York State. In the preceding eight years, he was Secretary of State of New York and then was elected Lieutenant Governor. His public career has been distinguished by numerous national addresses on critical domestic issues. He is the author of several books and the coeditor of *Lincoln on Democracy*.

The Honorable David N. Dinkins was Borough President of Manhattan for one term, and Clerk of the City of New York for a full decade before being elected as its 106th Mayor in 1989. He has also served as a State Assemblyman and as President of the New York City Board of Education.

Thomas P. Dowling, Esq. is the Vice Chairman of the New York State Public Health Council. He has also served as Co-Chairman of the Governor's Health Advisory Council for New York State. A nationally known patent lawyer, he is the Senior Partner of the Morgan & Finnegan law firm in New York.

John Duffy is Past President of the American Association of Medical Historians and is Professor Emeritus at both Tulane University and the University of Maryland. He is the author of the classic two-volume *History of Public Health in New York City* as well as the definitive record of American public health, *The Sanitarians.*

Marianne C. Fahs is Associate Professor of Economics and Community Health at the Mount Sinai School of Medicine in New York. She is the author of numerous articles and textbook chapters on cost-effectiveness and long-term health care.

Margaret C. Heagarty, M.D. is Director of Pediatrics at Harlem Hospital Center in New York. She is also Professor of Pediatrics at Columbia University's College of Physicians & Surgeons. She has been a member of numerous regional and national expert committees on child care.

The Honorable James Jones is the Chairman and Chief Executive Officer of the American Stock Exchange. For fourteen years, he was the Congressman from Oklahoma's 1st District, serving as Chairman of the House Budget Committee and the Social Security Committee. He is also the current Chairman of the American Business Conference, and is a director of numerous companies and public organizations.

The Honorable Charles Rangel represents the 16th Congressional District of New York. He has been a member of the House of Representatives since 1970. He is Chairman of the Select Committee on Narcotics Abuse and Control. He is also a senior member of the Ways and Means Committee.

David Rogers, M.D. is Chairman of both the New York City and New York State Panels on AIDS and is Vice Chairman of the national panel. He has also served as President of the Robert Wood Johnson Foundation, Dean of the Johns Hopkins Medical School, and is currently Walsh McDermott Professor of Medicine at Cornell University Medical School.

Deborah Steelman, Esq. is Chairman of the Advisory Council on Social Security. She has also served as Deputy Assistant to the President of the United States, as Associate Director of The Office of Management and Budget, and as Director of Domestic Policy for the Bush Presidential Campaign.

Stephen B. Thacker, M.D. is Director of Epidemiology Programs at the Department of Health & Human Services' Centers for Disease Control in Atlanta, Georgia. He is also the Editor in Chief of *Epidemiological Reviews*. He is on the public health and community medicine faculties of both Mount Sinai School of Medicine in New York and Emory University in Georgia.

Notes

Assuring Public Health in a Democracy:
A Historical Perspective

1. John M. Toner, "Boards of Health. . . ," selection from public health reports and papers presented at the meetings of the American Public Health Association (1873-1883), p. 499.

2. John Duffy, *A History of Public Health in New York City, 1625-1866* (New York: Russell Sage Foundation, 1968), pp. 42-45.

3. Ibid., pp. 101-05.

4. *Minutes of the Common Council of New York, 1675-1775* (New York, 1905), vol. II, pp. 481, 494-504; Duffy, *History of Public Health in New York City, 1625-1866*, pp. 134-37.

5. [New York] *Evening Post*, September 6-8, 1819.

6. *Address of the Board of Health of the City of New York to their Fellow Citizens* (New York, 1828); [New York] *Daily Tribune*, August 3, 4, 1849.

7. Duffy, *History of Public Health in New York City, 1625-1866*, pp. 546-70.

8. New York State Laws, 89th sess., chap. 74, February 26, 1866, pp. 114-44.

9. Minutes of the Metropolitan Board of Health, March 2-8, 1866, New York City Department of Health.

10. Duffy, *A History of Public Health in New York City, 1866-1966* (New York: Russell Sage Foundation, 1974), pp. 6-19.

11. Ibid., pp. 143-47.

12. Annual Report of the Board of Health of the City of New York, 1907, pp. 104-12; [New York] *Times*, June 29, July 1, 2, 10, August 7, November 24, 1907; [New York] *Tribune*, June 28-29, July 30, 1907.

13. Haven Emerson, "A Monograph on the Epidemic of Poliomyelitis (*Infantile Paralysis*) in New York City in 1916," *Public Health Monographs*, vol. II, pt. 2, no. 16 (New York, 1917), pp. 11-21; *Annual Report of the Board of Health, 1916*, pp. 24-25. "The Importance of the Present Epidemic of Poliomyelitis," July 13, 1916, manuscript, Haven Emerson Public Health Library, New York City (special stenographic report corrected by the author for *Archives of Pediatrics*), p. 589.

14. *Annual Report of the Board of Health, 1941-48*, pp. 44-45; Times, February 12-15, 19, March 5, 9, 12, 19, 1946; *Herald Tribune*, February 19, March 5, 12-13, 20, 1946; personal interview with Ernest L. Stebbins, January 27, 1972.

15. Duffy, *History of Public Health in New York City, 1866-1966*, pp. 154-58.

16. Fred L. Soper, *Ventures in World Health: The Memoirs of Fred Lowe Soper*, John Duffy, ed. (Washington, D.C.: Pan American World Health Organization, 1977), chaps. 7-10, 19, 20.

17. William H. Park, "Typhoid Bacilli Carriers," *Journal of the American Medical Association* 51 (1908), pp. 981-82; S. Josephine Baker, *Fighting for Life* (New York: MacMillan Co., 1939), pp. 72-76.

The Role of the Law in Public Health

1. Quoted in John Duffy, *A History of Public Health in New York City 1625-1866* (New York: Russell Sage Foundation, 1968) and citing Records of New Amsterdam VII, 187.

2. Inoculation against smallpox—practiced by abrading the skin of the treated individual and then introducing pus from a smallpox sore to the lesion—spread throughout the colonies during the eighteenth century, and is said to have originated in Asia. John Duffy, *Epidemics in Colonial America*, pp. 28-30.

3. Revised Laws, Chapter 75, §137.

4. The statute also provided that "Whoever, being over twenty-one years of age and not under guardianship refuses or neglects to comply with such requirement shall forfeit $5." 197 U.S. 1, 12; 25 Sup. Ct. Rep. 358, 359.

5. 197 U.S. 1, 12; 25 Sup. Ct. Rep. 358, 359.

6. 197 U.S. 1, 23; 25 Sup. Ct. Rep. 358, 360.

7. 197 U.S. 1 (1905), 25 Sup Ct Rep 358.

8. 197 U.S. 1, 25; 25 Sup. Ct. Rep. 358, 360.

9. Ibid.

10. 197 U.S. 1, 25; 25 Sup. Ct. Rep. 358, 361.

11. 197 U.S. at 25; 25 Sup. Ct. Rep. at 361.

12. Ibid.

13. 197 U.S. at 27; 25 Sup. Ct. Rep. at 362.

14. 197 U.S. at 34; 25 Sup. Ct. Rep. at 365.

15. 197 U.S. at 38; 25 Sup. Ct. Rep. at 366.

Suffer the Little Children: A View from the Trenches

1. Agenda for Children Tomorrow Implementation Project, *Community District Profile, Central Harlem, Manhattan 10*, July 1, 1991.

2. Greater New York March of Dimes/United Hospital Fund of New York, *Infants at Risk. Solutions Within Our Reach*, 1991.

3. For 1990: *Current Population Survey, 1991.* For 1966: Housing & Vacancy Survey, *Median Income for All Renter Households*, 1965.

4. For 1990-91: New York City Human Resources Administration, Office of Fiscal Operations. For 1966: Monthly Average, 1966, *Monthly Statistical Report*, July 1966.

5. New York State Department of Social Services, *Statistical Supplement*; DA&R *Fact Sheet*.

6. New York City Human Resources Administration, Crisis Intervention Services, "Emergency Housing Services for Homeless Families," *Monthly Report*, June 1991.

7. "The Measles Emergency," City Health Information, vol. 10, no. 3, May 1991.

The Economic Consequences of Inaction

1. U.S. Bureau of the Census, U.S. Census of Population; 1960 and 1970; 1980 Census of Population, vol 1, chap. A (PC80-1-A) and Supplementary Report, Metropolitan Statistical Areas (PC80-81S1-18); Current Population Reports, Series P-26, No. 85-AL-C to 85-WY-C and Series P-25, No 1039.

2. Estimates in this discussion are derived from studies of the cost of illness by D. P. Rice, T. A. Hodgson, and A. N. Kopstein, "The economic costs of illness: A replication and update," *Health Care Financing Review*, Fall 1985, pp. 61-80. Figures for 1991 are estimated by applying the prior seventeen-year average annual indirect cost growth rate to 1985 cost estimates and updating the dollar values to 1991 dollars using the consumer price index.

3. J. E. Osborne, "AIDS and Public Policy," *AIDS* 3 (supplement 1), 1989, pp. S 297-300.

4. A. A. Scitovsky, "The Economic Impact of AIDS," *Health Affairs*, Fall 1988, pp. 32-45.

5. Estimates in this discussion are derived from the study by Scitovsky, "The Economic Impact of AIDS," pp. 32-45, using the proportion of total U.S. AIDS cases that are in New York State and New York City, according to data from U.S. Department of Health and Human Services, Centers for Disease Control, *HIV/AIDS Surveillance Report*, July 1991, pp. 1-18.

6. P. Passell, "Forces in Society, and Reaganism, Helped Dig Deeper Hole for Poor," *The New York Times*, July 16, 1989, p. A1.

7. Office of Policy and Financial Management, Human Resources Administration, The City of New York, unpublished data, July 1991.

8. Ibid.

9. U.S. Bureau of the Census, "Current Population Survey for New York City," Average of 1985-86 estimates of percent of population living in poverty. National data from Current Population Report, Series P-60, #158.

10. T. Smeeding, B. B. Torrey, and M. Rein, "Patterns of Income and Poverty: The Economic Status of Children and the Elderly in Eight Countries," in J. L. Palmer, T. Smeeding, and B. B. Torrey, eds., *The Vulnerable* (Washington, D.C.: The Urban Institute Press, 1988), pp. 89-119.

11. U.S. Bureau of the Census, "Current Population Survey for New York City," Average of 1985-86 estimates of percent of population living in poverty. National data from Current Population Report, Series P-60, #158.

12. H. E. Sigerist, *Medicine and Human Welfare* (College Park, Maryland: McGrath Publishing Co., 1970).

13. "Health Status of the Disadvantaged, Chartbook 1986." DHHS Publication No. (HRSA) HRS-P-DV86-2 (Washington, D.C.: U.S. Government Printing Office, 1986).

14. U.S. Department of Health and Human Services, Centers for Disease Control, *Strategic plan for the elimination of childhood lead poisoning*, February 1991, pp. 1-53.

15. Ibid.

16. Ibid.

17. P. Levi, *The Periodic Table*, 1st American edition (New York: Schocken Books, 1984).

18. The National Commission to Prevent Infant Mortality, *Troubling Trends: The Health of America's Next Generation*, February 1990.

19. U.S. Congress, Office of Technology Assessment, *Healthy Children: Investing in the Future*, OTA-H-345 (Washington, D.C.: U.S. Government Printing Office, 1988).

20. The National Commission to Prevent Infant Mortality, *Troubling Trends: The Health of America's Next Generation*, February 1990.

21. A. B. Bloch, W. A. Orenstein, H. C. Stetler, et al., "Health Impact of Measles Vaccination in the United States," *Pediatrics* vol. 76, 1985, pp. 524-32.

22. C. C. White, J. P. Koplan, and W. A. Orenstein, "Benefits, risks and costs of immunization for measles, mumps and rubella," *American Journal of Public Health* vol. 75, no. 7, 1985, pp. 739-44.

23. A. R. Hinman and J. P. Koplan, "Pertussis and Pertussis Vaccine: Reanalysis of Benefits, Risks, and Costs," *JAMA* 251, 1984, pp. 3109-13.

24. *The State of the World's Children* (New York: UNICEF, 1987).

25. J. Mason, *The Nation's Health* (newsletter of the American Public Health Association), August 1991.

26. J. S. Mandelblatt and M. C. Fahs, "The cost-effectiveness of cervical cancer screening for low-income elderly women," *Journal of the American Medical Association* vol. 259, no. 16, 1988, pp. 2409-13.

27. Health Care Financing Administration, Division of National Cost Estimates, U.S. Department of Health and Human Services, 1989.

28. R. J. Blendon and K. Donelan, "Interpreting public opinion surveys," *Health Affairs* vol.10, no. 2, Summer 1991, pp. 166-69.

29. M. Freudenheim, "Job Growth in Health Care Soars," *The New York Times*, March 5, 1990.

30. Ibid. Also, K. R. Levit, H. C. Lazenby, S. W. Letsch, and C. A. Cowan, "National health care spending, 1989," *Health Affairs*, vol. 10, no. 1, Spring 1991, pp. 117-30.

31. U. E. Reinhardt, "Health care spending and American competitiveness," *Health Affairs*, vol. 8, no. 4, Winter 1989, pp. 5-21.

32. Ibid.

33. Ibid.

34. Ibid. Also, V. R. Fuchs, "The health sector's share of the gross national product," *Science* vol. 246, 1990, pp. 534-38.

35. U. E. Reinhardt, "Health care spending and American competitiveness," *Health Affairs*, vol. 8, no. 4, Winter 1989, pp. 5-21.

36. Ibid.

37. Ibid.

38. Organization for Economic Cooperation and Development Secretariat, "Health care expenditure and other data," *Health Care Financing Review*, 1989 Annual

Supplement, Baltimore, MD. U.S. Department of Health and Human Services, December 1989.

39. M. I. Roemer, R. Roemer, "Global health, national development and the role of government," *American Journal of Public Health*, vol. 80, no. 10, October 1990, pp. 1188-92.

40. Ibid.

41. S. Cereseto and H. Waitzkin, "Economic development, political-economic system, and the physical quality of life," *Journal of Public Health Policy*, Spring 1988, pp. 104-20.

42. G. J. Schieber, J-P. Poullier, "International health spending: Issues and trends," *Health Affairs*, vol. 10, no. 1, Spring 1991, pp. 106-16.

43. U.S. Department of State, Bureau of Intelligence and Research, "Economic Growth of IECD Countries, 1978-1988," Report No. IRR 205 (revised), 1989, and unpublished data.

44. J. Hadley, *More Medical Care, Better Health?* (Washington, D.C.: The Urban Institute Press, 1982).

45. R. Heilbroner, "Economic Predictions," *New Yorker*, July 8, 1991.

46. J. Hadley, J. Holahan, and W. Scanlon, "Can fee-for-service reimbursement coexist with demand creation?" *Inquiry*, vol. 16, 1979, p. 247. Also, T. Rice, "The impact of changing medicare reimbursement rates on physician-induced demand," *Medical Care*, vol. 21, 1983, p. 803. Also, L. F. Rossiter and G. R. Wilensky, "A reexamination of the use of physician services: The role of the physician-initiated demand," *Inquiry*, 1983, p. 162. Also, M. C. Fahs, "Physician response to the United Mine Workers cost sharing program: The other side of the coin," *Health Services Research*, forthcoming.

47. K. R. Levit, H. C. Lazenby, S. W. Letsch, and C. A. Cowan, "National health care spending, 1989," *Health Affairs*, vol. 10, no. 1, Spring 1991, pp. 117-30.

48. P. R. Lee and L. Etheredge, "Clinical Freedom: Two Lessons for the U.K. from U.S. Experience with Privatisation of Health Care," *The Lancet*, February 4, 1989, pp. 263-65.

49. P. J. Cunningham, A. C. Monheit, "Insuring the children: A decade of change," *Health Affairs*, vol. 9, no. 4, 1990, pp. 76-90.

50. Ibid.

51. Ibid.

52. S. Woolhandler and D. U. Himmelstein, "The Deteriorating Administrative Efficiency of the U.S. Health Care System," *The New England Journal of Medicine*, vol. 324, no. 18, 1991, pp. 1253-58.

53. Ibid.

54. J. Hadley, E. P. Steinberg, and J. Feder, "Comparison of Uninsured and Privately Insured Hospital Patients: Condition on Admission, Resource Use, and Outcome," *JAMA*, vol. 265, no. 3, 1991, pp. 374-79.

55. K. Davis, "Expanded Use of Community Health Centers: Potential Savings to Medicaid," Paper prepared for 1981 Commonwealth Fund Forum, "Medical Care for the Poor: What Can States Do in the 1980's?" Philadelphia, Pennsylvania,

August 9-12, 1981. Also, U.S. General Accounting Office, Report to the Chairman, Committee on Government Operations, House of Representatives, *Canadian Health Insurance: Lessons for the United States*, GAO/ HDR-91-90, June 1991.

56. U.S. General Accounting Office, Report to the Chairman, Committee on Government Operations, House of Representatives, *Canadian Health Insurance: Lessons for the United States*, GAO/HDR-91-90, June 1991.

57. M. Grossman, *Health Benefits of Increases in Alcohol and Cigarette Taxes*, National Bureau of Economic Research, Reprint No. 1414, Cambridge, Massachusetts.

58. Ibid.

59. K. W. Deuschle and F. Eberson, "Community medicine comes of age," *The Journal of Medical Education*, vol. 48, no. 12, 1968, pp. 1229-37.

A War Room for Health

1. R. Wallace, "Urban Decertification, Public Health and Public Order: `Planned Shrinkage,' Violent Death, Substance Abuse and AIDS in the Bronx," *Social Science and Medicine*, vol. 31, 1990, pp. 801-13.

2. E. Rosenthal, "Health Problems of Inner City Poor Reach Crisis Point," *The New York Times*, December 24, 1990.

3. C. McCord, and H. P. Freeman, "Excess Mortality in Harlem," *New England Journal of Medicine*, vol. 322, January 18, 1990, pp. 173-77.

4. J. Dixon and H. G. Welch, "Priority Setting: Lessons from Oregon," *Lancet*, vol. 1, April 13, 1991, pp. 891-94.